Diagnosis and Treatment
of
Low Back Pain

Diagnosis and Treatment
of
Low Back Pain

Neil Kahanovitz, M.D.

Executive Director, National Spine Center,
Anderson Clinic, Arlington, Virginia, and
Clinical Associate Professor of Orthopedic Surgery,
Georgetown University Medical Center, Washington, D.C.

Raven Press 🦅 New York

Raven Press Ltd., 1185 Avenue of the Americas, New York, New York, 10036

Made in the United States of America

Library of Congress Cataloging-in-Publication Data

Kahanovitz, Neil.
    Diagnosis and treatment of low back pain / Neil Kahanovitz.
        p.   cm.
    Includes index.
    ISBN 0-88167-775-2
    1. Backache. I. Title.
    [DNLM: 1. Backache—diagnosis. 2. Backache—therapy. WE 755
K12d]
    RD771.B217K46   1991
    617.5′64—dc20
    DLC
    for Library of Congress   91-12322
                                                                        CIP

The material contained in this volume was submitted as previously upublished material, except in the instances in which credit has been given to the source from which some of the illustrative material was derived.

Great care has been taken to maintain the accuracy of the information contained in the volume. However, neither Raven Press nor the editors can be held responsible for errors or for any consequences arising from the use of the information contained herein.

9 8 7 6 5 4 3 2 1

To Melanie, Alexia, and Kate
for their patience and understanding

Contents

Preface

As an orthopedic resident, if given the choice of taking weekend call or covering the low back clinic, I would have invariably chosen call. Nothing could be worse than listening to patients complain about chronic low back pain, refilling narcotic pain prescriptions, and filling out disability forms. Not until years later did I realize that taking care of patients with low back pain could be less painful than the back pain itself.

This book is primarily intended for those physicians and therapists who perceive the low back pain patient negatively, as I and many others have in the past. I hope that, after reading this book, these individuals will be able to care for the low back pain patient with a fresh and, more important, an objective approach that simplifies much of the confusion and anxiety provoked by the low back pain patient.

Neil Kahanovitz, M.D.

Acknowledgments

This book would have never been possible, without the help of many people along the way. Thanks go to Dr. Paul Johanson for his support and guidance during my residency. A special "Thank you" is owed to Dr. David Levine for involving me in the world of spinal surgery through his endless enthusiasm, encouragement, and friendship.

Shawna Knauer and Lisa Bragg deserve a great deal of credit for their often thankless hours of help and support. Mary Rogers deserves my gratitude for giving me the opportunity to write this book as well as her help along the way. I would also like to thank Donna Cavi for her skillful illustrations and, last but not least, my partners at the Anderson Clinic for their support.

Neil Kahanovitz, M.D.

Diagnosis and Treatment
of
Low Back Pain

1
Epidemiology

Low back pain is so prevalent in our population that one wonders whether it is truly abnormal to experience low back pain. Perhaps the 20–30% of the adult population who will never have low back pain are the pathologic group since the large majority of the adults in the Western world experience low back pain at least once in their adult lives. At least 70–80% of all Americans will experience low back pain of varying intensity that will affect their daily activities during their adult lives. Thus the vast majority of adults will be affected by these annoying and often disabling symptoms. Fortunately, very few of us will have prolonged symptoms that will leave us permanently disabled or in chronic pain.

For many physicians, the most interesting aspects of treating lumbar spine disease are the surgical procedures used to alleviate low back and sciatic pain. However, only a fraction of all patients with low back pain ultimately need surgical intervention. In fact, only 1–2% of all patients experiencing low back pain who are seen by a physician will be candidates for any type of surgical procedure. This contrasts sharply with the lifetime prevalence of low back pain that ranges from 13.8–31% (1,4). Therefore it is easy to see that much of our interest and focus on the treatment of patients with low back pain must shift from surgical to nonsurgical means. This has become more and more evident despite our fascination with the ability to cure back and sciatic pain with an ever-increasing variety of surgical procedures.

Most patients experience their first bout of low back pain during the third decade of their lives. However, the prevalence of low back pain increases from the third decade until it peaks in the 55–64 year-old range. After age 65, the prevalence of low back pain continues to decrease (1,2).

When patients are questioned as to the severity of their pain, there is usually no consistency in their responses. There appears to be an almost even distribution of those reporting mild, moderate, or severe low back pain except for a slight preponderance of those patients reporting moderate to severe pain during their first episode. In contrast, there is evidence that the severity of pain at the onset of the patient's symptoms increases with the increasing age of the patient at the first onset of low back pain (1). Unfortunately there does not appear to be any rational physiologic explanation for this.

Probably the first and foremost clinical as well as therapeutic differentiation is the separation of those patients presenting with low back pain from those patients presenting with sciatica with or without low back pain. The incidence of patients presenting with sciatica is far less than the incidence of those with low back pain alone. Of all the patients presenting with low back pain, only 10–12% will have concomitant sciatica. However, those patients with *severe* low back pain more commonly have associated sciatica than do those with more mild to moderate low back pain. The peak age for the onset of sciatic pain is somewhat later than for the onset of low pack pain alone, and it occurs in the 45–54-year-old age range (1). Of those patients with sciatic symptoms, only 1–2% will ever require surgical intervention. Clearly, only a small minority of patients having sciatic symptoms warrant surgical intervention.

Despite the small number of patients requiring surgery, the impact of low back pain on modern society cannot be minimized. For all workers in the United States under the age of 45, low back pain is the leading cause of lost productivity and lost time from work. In fact, low back pain is the costliest of all the musculoskeletal ailments to the American medical system. In 1986 alone, over 5 million people were unable to work due to disabling low back symptoms. In total, there were 11 million people treated for low back impairments that year (3). The spiraling costs are staggering when we take into account the enormous financial drain of lost productivity and time lost from work, diagnostic and treatment modalities, and litigation and disability claims. Recent estimates range from a low of $18 billion to a high of $50 billion annually.

These figures seem inordinately high for what at first glance appears for the majority of patients to be a benign self-limited ailment. It is interesting that, after 6 months, roughly 7% of all patients with low pain will still continue to have symptoms, and, by 1 year, only 2% will still complain of symptoms. However, those 7% of patients who still have pain 6 months after the onset of symptoms will consume over 85–90% of all the money spent on the treatment and compensation of low back pain. A Canadian study found in 1981 that 75% of all money spent on low back compensation costs was spent on only the 7% of patients with a spinal disorder who had been absent from work for more than 6 months (3).

These facts and figures are not surprising when we realize that low back pain is such a common ailment that affects almost 80% of all adults in the United States. It is startling to realize the enormous impact that it has on the cost to society for the diagnosis, treatment, lost productivity, and compensation for what outwardly appears to be a rather straightforward clinical problem. Unfortunately, as we will see throughout this book, diagnosis and treatment of patients with low back pain must deal not only with the objective signs and symptoms of lumbar spine disease, but also the complicated and often confusing psychosocial and economic factors that play heavily on the physician's ability to properly diagnose and treat patients with low back pain.

A large part of the physician's ability to diagnose and treat patients with lumbar spine disease will depend on his or her ability to identify the true objective signs and symptoms necessary to accurately treat the patient with low back pain. It will quickly become apparent that the successful treatment of patients with low back pain is heavily dependent on timely diagnosis and the institution of appropriate treatment methods. Only the proper diagnosis and treatment will prevent these patients from becoming one of those 7% of patients with low back pain who become a burden on our society and medical system.

REFERENCES

1. Deyo RA, Tsui-Wu YJ: Descriptive epidemiology of low back pain and its related medical care in the United States. *Spine* 1987;12:264–268.
2. Lavsky-Shulan M, Wallace RB, Kohout FJ, Lewke JH, Morris MC, Smith IM: Prevalence and functional correlates of low back pain in the elderly: the Iowa 65 + Rural Health Study. *J Am Geriatr Soc* 1985;33:23–28.
3. Spitzer WO, et al: Scientific approach to the assessment and management of activity-related spinal disorders. *Spine* 1987;12:75.
4. Svensson HO, Nedin A, Wilhelmsson C, et al: Low-back pain in relation to other diseases and cardiovascular risk factors. *Spine* 1983;8:277–285.

2

Anatomy

It is often impossible to identify the exact etiologic abnormality responsible for low back pain. This is one of the most frustrating aspects of treating patients with low back pain. For the majority of patients, there will be no anatomic structure that one can palpate or point to on a radiograph and definitively tell the patient "This is where your pain is coming from." Despite an endless supply of theoretic explanations of the possible etiologies responsible for the common "garden variety" types of low back pain, there is no consensus concerning which anatomic structure, physiologic abnormality, or biomechanical alteration is responsible for the pain.

A large majority of these theoretic explanations are simply justifications for proposed treatment modalities for symptomatic patients. These modalities range from trigger point and facet injections to dorsal root rhizotomies to a variety of fusion techniques. So far, few have been scientifically proved to have a true therapeutic benefit for the majority of patients with low back pain.

Despite this rather gloomy introduction, an understanding of the normal anatomy and the degenerative changes associated with the normal aging process will give the treating physician a solid foundation upon which to base not only diagnostic and therapeutic but also surgical recommendations. Just as important, the physician may now realize which conservative and surgical treatment modalities have no valid anatomic or physiologic basis for their use.

There are normally five lumbar vertebrae. On occasion there may be an additional vertebra that may be either partially sacralized or a sacral vertebra so-called *lumbarized*. (Fig. 2–1) There is no universal agreement on the definition of a vertebra's being sacralized or lumbarized. So it is best to identify the last truly mobile or articulating segment as the *last mobile segment* (LMS). This will avoid any confusion between the radiologist and surgeon when attempting to communicate a possible anatomic abnormality.

The lumbar vertebrae are the largest vertebrae in the body. They continue to increase in size from cephalad to caudad. The same holds for the size of the intervening intervertebral discs, except that the L4–5 disc is typically the largest, and the L5–S1 disc is usually smaller (Fig. 2–2). As the size of the

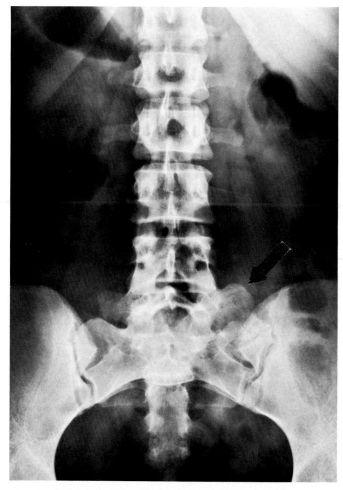

FIG. 2–1. Note the sacralization of the last lumbar vertebra with the enlarged spinous process. To avoid confusion, this segment should be referred to as the *last mobile segment.*

vertebrae increases, so does the size of the spinal canal. Interpedicular distance and cross-sectional diameter characteristically increase from L1 through L5. (Fig. 2–3) A variety of hereditary conditions (the best known of these being achondroplasia) are characterized by decreasing proximal to caudad spinal canal diameter and pedicular height.

Articulation of the individual vertebra occurs posteriorly between the two facets and anteriorly with the intervertebral disc. Each intervertebral disc is referred to by its proximal and distal vertebra, i.e., the L4–5 or L3–4 disc. The normal alignment of the lumbar spine in the sagittal plane is lordotic.

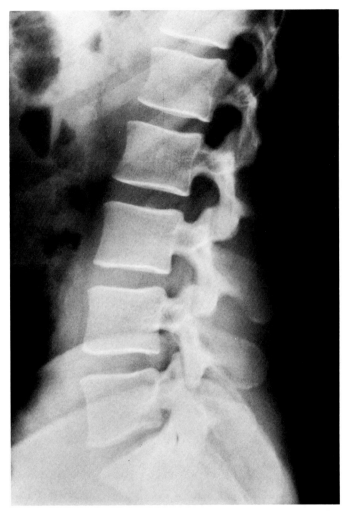

FIG. 2–2. The lumbar disc spaces continue to increase in size until the L4–5 disc, which is typically the largest. The L5–S1 disc is almost always smaller than the L4–5 disc.

The lordosis balances the normal thoracic kyphosis and effectively maintains the head and trunk over the body's center of gravity.

It is extremely important to realize that any motion involving the lumbar vertebrae must take into account the motion of all three articulations: the two posterior facet joint complexes and the anterior intervertebral disc articulation (Fig. 2–4). To best understand the interdependent relationship of the posterior and anterior structures, it is easiest to view the anatomic unit of motion as the motion segment. The motion segment consists of the superior

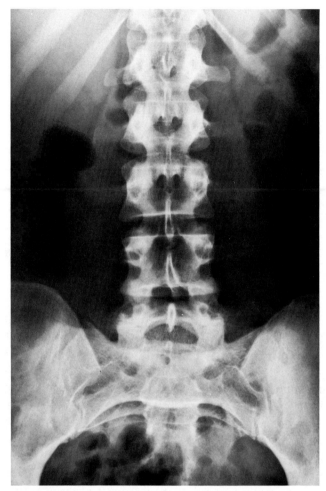

FIG. 2–3. The interpedicular distance and width of the spinal canal increases from cephalad to caudad. Note the significantly wider canal diameter at L5 compared to L1 or L2.

vertebra with its articulating inferior facets, the intervening intervertebral disc, and an inferior vertebra with its articulating superior facet joints (Fig. 2–4).

In addition to these articulations, there are a number of ligamentous structures that also connect the adjacent vertebra of the motion segment (Fig. 2–5). The most posterior ligamentous structure is the supraspinous ligament connecting the most posterior portion of the spinous processes. Anterior to the supraspinous ligament is the interspinous ligament that connects the majority of the spinous process until it meets the ligamentum flavum anteriorly.

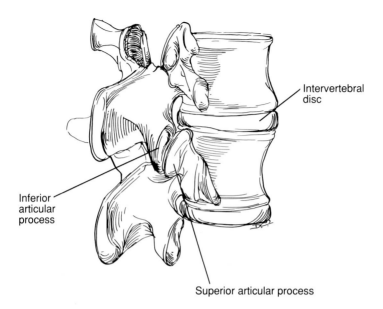

FIG. 2–4. The motion of the motion segment involves the posterior facet joints as well as the anterior intervetebral disc. All three articulations must be taken into account when discussing the motion of the motion segment.

The ligamentum flavum is a highly specialized ligamentous structure that contains elastin. Throughout life, the elastin allows for elasticity of this ligament. The ligamentum flavum arises from the superior margin of the inferior vertebra and attaches in a fan-like distribution to the distal half of the underside of the superior vertebra (Fig. 2–6). Normally there is a small cleft in the midline separating right and left sides. As the ligamentum flavum fans out proximally to attach to the underside of the proximal vertebra, it also fans out laterally to form the undersurface of the facet joint. There is no true fibrous facet joint capsule present anteriorly but only the ligamentum flavum forming the anterior facet joint capsule (Fig. 2–7).

The posterior floor of the spinal canal is formed by the thin posterior longitudinal ligament. Immediately anterior to this flimsy ligament are the outermost layers of the annulus fibrosis of the intervertebral disc. The most anterior structure of the spinal column is the anterior longitudinal ligament. This ligament is much thicker and stronger than the posterior longitudinal ligament and contributes a great deal more to the stability of the spinal column than its posterior counterpart (Fig. 2–8).

The articular facets are unique to the lumbar spine. At the junction of the pedicle, transverse process, and lamina, the pars interarticularis gives rise to the superior and inferior facets. The concave superior facet is directed poste-

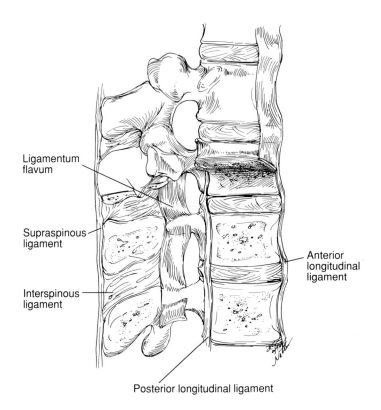

Ligamentum
flavum

Supraspinous
ligament

Interspinous
ligament

Anterior
longitudinal
ligament

Posterior longitudinal ligament

FIG. 2–5. In addition to the facet joint and disc articulations, the adjacent
vertebrae are linked by anterior and posterior ligamentous structures.

riorly and medially, while the inferior facet is directed more anteriorly and
laterally (Fig. 2–9). The posterior capsule is formed by a typical fibrous
joint capsule. The anterior portion of the facet joint capsule is formed by the
ligamentum flavum.

The unique orientation of the facet joint complex in the lumbar spine
allows for virtually no rotation. Clinical measurements have found that motion in the sagittal plane allows for an average of 55 degrees of flexion and
25 degrees of extension. In addition to flexion and extension, there are approximately 45 degrees of lateral bending of the spine between L1 and S1.

The intervertebral disc is a complex anatomic and biomechanical structure that is attached to the vertebral body endplates by the outer fibers of the
annulus fibrosus, or Sharpey's fibers. The annulus fibrosis is made up of
concentric layers of collagen that encircle the anatomically distinctive nucleus pulposus (Fig. 2–10). There is a gradual transition between the nu-

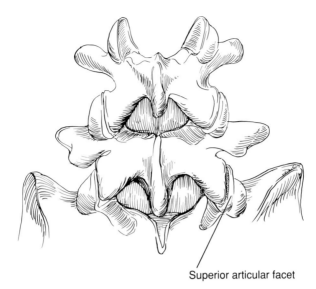

Superior articular facet

FIG. 2–6. The ligamentum flavum arises from the superior laminar edge of the inferior vertebra and attaches in a fan-like distribution to the anterior or undersurface of the distal half of the superior vertebral lamina. The lateral expansion of the ligamentum flavum forms the anterior capsule of the facet joint.

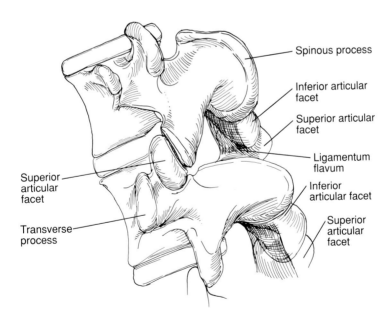

Spinous process

Inferior articular facet

Superior articular facet

Ligamentum flavum

Inferior articular facet

Superior articular facet

Superior articular facet

Transverse process

FIG. 2–7. The lateral extension of the ligamentum flavum forms the anterior facet joint capsule. This lateral portion of the ligamentum flavum also forms the posterior roof of the lateral recess.

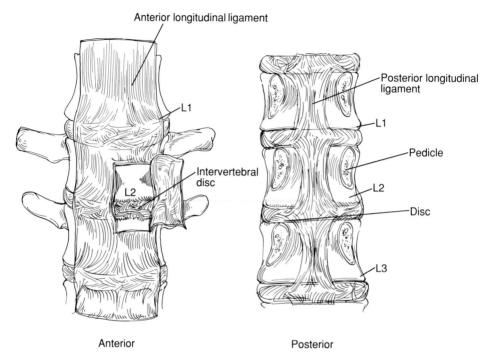

Anterior longitudinal ligament

Posterior longitudinal
ligament

L1

L1

Intervertebral
disc

Pedicle

L2

L2

Disc

L3

Anterior   Posterior

FIG. 2–8. Posteriorly, the vertebral body is covered by the flimsy posterior longitudinal ligament in the spinal canal. Anteriorly, the anterior longitudinal ligament provides significantly more structural integrity than the posterior longitudinal ligament.

cleus and annulus with no clearcut anatomic or histologic boundaries separating the two structures. Unlike the annulus, the majority of the nucleus is made up of a variety of mucopolysaccharides produced by the cells interspersed throughout the nucleus.

The intervertebral lumbar disc does not have a direct blood supply. However, one should not mistake the intervertebral disc as metabolically inactive. By means of diffusion through the cartilaginous endplates, there is active metabolic activity in both the nucleus and the annulus.

The biomechanical function of the intervertebral disc has frequently been described as an anatomic shock absorber. Because of its unique structure, the intervertebral disc is able to protect the less forgiving bony vertebrae from forces that would normally result in failure of the bone and ultimate vertebral fracture.

Intradiscal pressure varies with the applied load. Although there is also load sharing by the facet joints, the paraspinal muscles, and the intra-abdominal pressure, the majority of force transmitted through the spinal canal is counteracted by the intervertebral disc. The classic study of intradiscal

A

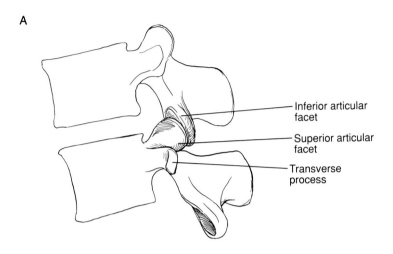

Inferior articular
facet

Superior articular
facet

Transverse
process

B

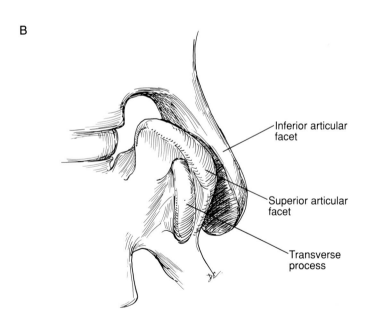

Inferior articular
facet

Superior articular
facet

Transverse
process

FIG. 2–9. The sagitally oriented superior (**A**) and inferior facet (**B**) joints readily allow flexion and extension. Their unique orientations are significantly different from those of either the cervical or thoracic facet joints.

pressure measurement was done by Nachemson in 1966 (1). A pressure transducer was inserted into the L3 disc of human volunteers. Measurements were recorded for various changes in position and activity. Among a variety of activities, standing in the erect position produced the least load of approximately 100 kg on the disc. This load progressively increased to 300 kg when the subject was sitting and lifting a 50 kg weight. This apparently avascular and simple structure has the unique capacity of dissipating loads that could not normally be tolerated by the bony vertebral column.

The sacrum, which articulates with the L5 vertebra, is formed by the fusion of five sacral vertebrae. Laterally, the alae project from the sacrum. Arising from the alae are the sacral articular facets that articulate with the inferior facets of L5 (Fig. 2–11). Since the sacrum is formed by five fused vertebrae, there are four ventral and dorsal neural foraminae that allow passage of the larger ventral sacral nerve roots and the smaller dorsal nerve roots.

The spinal cord ends at the L1–L2 level as the conus medullaris. Distally the intrathecal contents are made up of the cauda equina. At each vertebral level, a ventral and dorsal root unite to form the segmental nerve root. Each lumbar nerve root is identified by the pedicle adjacent to its exit through the intervertebral foramen (Fig. 2–12). For example the nerve root that exists just inferior to the L5 pedicle is the L5 nerve root.

As the nerve root exits the spine, it is contained in an anatomic space known as the *lateral recess* (Fig. 2–13). Proximally, the lateral recess is bound posteriorly and laterally by the most lateral portion of the lamina and its transition into the pars. At this level, the floor of the lateral recess is formed by the intervertebral disc. Just distally, the medially oriented supe-

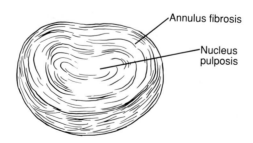

FIG. 2–10. Unlike the common misrepresentation of the intervertebral disc as two distinct entities comprised of an outer annulus and an inner circumscribed nucleus much like a jelly doughnut, the true disc anatomy is represented by a gradual transition of collagenous annular layers to the inner nuclear material comprised primarily of mucopolysaccharides.

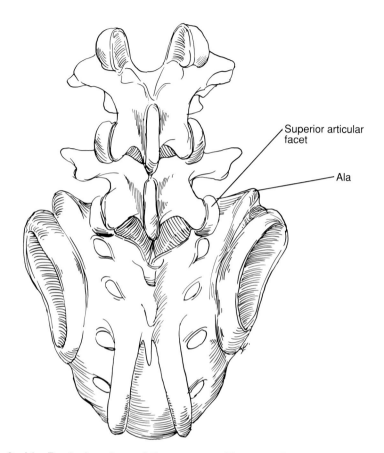

FIG. 2–11. Posterior view of the sacrum. Four small dorsal roots emerge from the dorsal foramen.

rior facet and its underlying coverage of ligamentum flavum comprise the posterior boundary of the lateral recess. The lateral border is formed by the pedicle and the floor is formed by the posterior aspect of the vertebral body. As the nerve root exits the spine, it passes close by and just inferior to the pedicle on its way out through the neural foramen.

The neural foramen is often confused with the lateral recess. It is best to think of the neural foramen as an anatomic plane or door through which the nerve root exits from the most lateral aspect of the spinal canal. Likewise, the lateral recess should be viewed as the tunnel or canal through which the nerve root travels just prior to its exit from the spinal canal through the neural foramen. Just distal to the pedicle, the dorsal root ganglion is located.

Normally, there is ample room for the nerve root in the lateral recess and neural foramen with no bony or ligamentous impingement. However, once

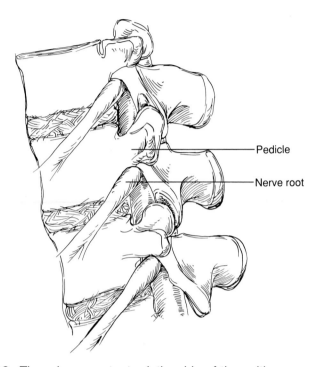

FIG. 2–12. There is a constant relationship of the exiting nerve root to the pedicle. Even in the presence of distorted anatomy and compressed nerve roots due to degenerative changes, the relationship of the nerve root to the pedicle remains constant and will often facilitate the location of the nerve root in difficult surgical cases.

the degenerative process begins, this space often becomes compromised. Understanding this phenomenon is, in fact, the key to understanding both the normal anatomy of aging as well as many of the pathophysiologic conditions that may accompany these degenerative changes.

With increasing age and usually by the fourth decade, intrinsic changes begin taking place within the intervertebral disc. The unique ability of the mucopolysaccharides contained in the nucleus pulposus begin to lose their ability to bind water molecules. In a sense, this causes the nuclear material to dessicate, thereby allowing the internal pressure of the nucleus to decrease. At the same time, fissures begin to appear in the nucleus as the result of the degeneration and necrosis taking place.

Similar degenerative changes are also occurring in the annulus fibrosis. Myxomatous degeneration and subsequent cystic formation disrupt the normal orderly architecture of the concentric annular fibers. Following these degenerative changes, collagenous fiber bundles begin to swell and sepa-

A

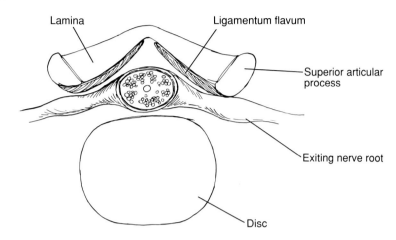

Lamina
Ligamentum flavum
Superior articular process
Exiting nerve root
Disc

B

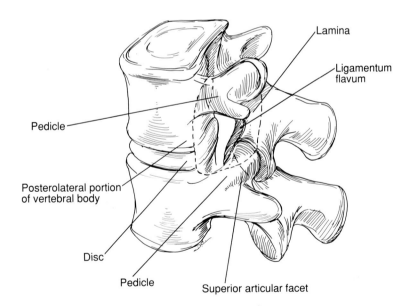

Lamina
Ligamentum flavum
Pedicle
Posterolateral portion of vertebral body
Disc
Pedicle
Superior articular facet

FIG. 2–13. The lateral recess is the tunnel or canal through which the nerve root travels on its way to the foramen (**A**). In the lateral recess the nerve root is susceptible to compression by a wide variety of anatomic structures that may be involved with degenerative disease. (**B**) Boundaries of the lateral recess.

rate. This ultimately leads to reversal patterns of the normal convex pattern of the annular fibers. Along with the reversed order of the annulus, actual ruptures of the annular fibers may also occur.

With these normal histologic and anatomic changes in the intervertebral disc comes a slowly progressive loss of intervertebral disc height. This is not an isolated physiologic event but, rather, it has great impact on virtually all other anatomic structures making up the lumbar motion segment.

As the disc space narrows, the most posterior annular fibers and posterior longitudinal ligament tend to bulge posteriorly into the spinal canal creating an anterior segmental bulging. At the same time, the facet joints begin to show progressive settling and subluxation due to the concomitant loss of anterior disc height (Fig. 2–14).

It is important to remember that all of the vertebral structures are interdependent. Any alteration in function of the anterior or posterior structures

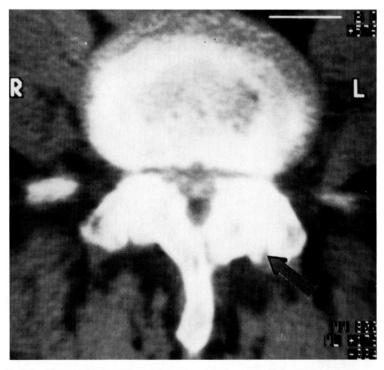

FIG. 2–14. Computerized tomography (CT) scan illustrating the progressive degenerative facet changes due to the altered facet joint mechanics concurrent with anterior disc space narrowing. As the disc narrows anteriorly, abnormal facet joint motion and stresses lead to hypertrophic spurring (arrow), subsequent lateral recess, and central spinal canal stenosis.

will affect the other in its normal physiologic function. Continued narrowing of the intervertebral disc anteriorly causes increasing subluxation and altered joint mechanics of the facet joints posteriorly (Fig. 2–15).

As this occurs, degenerative osteoarthritic changes begin to develop in the facet joints. The most structurally significant changes are the osteoarthritic spurs that form at the margins of the superior facets. Keeping in mind the ligamentum flavum's elastic properties, one can see that, as the intervertebral space narrows, the ligamentum flavum tends to buckle or fold inward into the spinal canal (Fig. 2–16). This is particularly important in the lateral recess where the ligamentum flavum forms the anterior capsule of the facet joint. In combination with the arthritic spurring of the superior facet and the infolded or apparently thickened ligamentum flavum, significant narrowing or compromise of the lateral recess may occur. It is easy, then, to anatomically visualize the phenomenon of lateral recess stenosis as this process continues (Fig. 2–17).

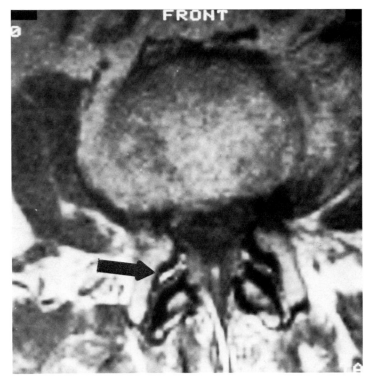

FIG. 2–15. Magnetic resonance imaging (MRI) demonstrating the subluxation of the facet joints (arrow) that occur in conjunction with the degeneration of the anterior structures of the motion segment.

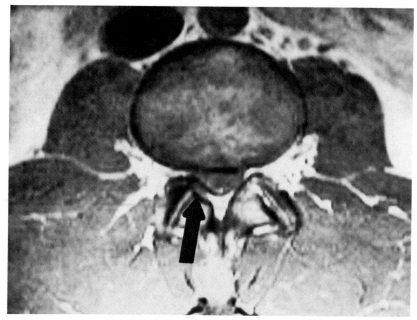

FIG. 2–16. As subluxation of the joints increases, the ligamentum flavum buckles into and impinges first upon the nerve root exiting the lateral recess and then into the central canal (*arrow*).

As this degenerative process continues, the more the posteromedial ligamentum flavum begins to encroach upon the spinal canal contents at its proximal attachment to the underside of the superior lamina. The ligamentum flavum slowly buckles inward as the disc space anteriorly continues to degenerate and narrow (Fig. 2–18). At the same time anteriorly, there is additional canal compromise by the increasingly bulging disc and laterally by the subluxated and degenerative facet joints. Thus, in the more advanced stage of degenerative change, it is quite easy to understand how these physiologic and anatomic changes result not only in lateral recess stenosis but also in central spinal canal stenosis as well. Although the degenerative changes responsible for lateral recess stenosis may be found as early as the late forties or fifties, central spinal canal stenosis is usually a rather slow process and does not normally begin until the seventh or eighth decade.

With these apparently simple anatomic and physiologic events taking place, it appears that it would be a rather straightforward process to pinpoint the exact painful anatomical abnormality. Even though these anatomic alterations appear straightforward, the exact etiology of spinal pain remains elu-

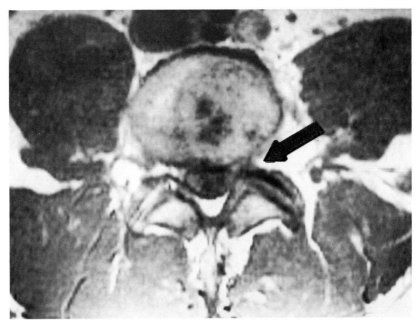

FIG. 2–17. Note the asymmetrical narrowing of the lateral recess (*arrow*). In combination with the lateral bulging disc, there is marked compromise of the space available for the exiting nerve root.

sive. Despite extensive research, both clinical and experimental, no clearcut etiology explaining what actually causes the pain has emerged. A number of theories propose the musculature, facet joint, internal disc disruption, facet joint capsule, and synovium as the cause of pain, but none have been scientifically or definitively proved to be the responsible etiologic agent for even the most simple presentation of low back pain.

Sciatic pain would appear to be much easier to explain on a physiologic and anatomic basis. Unfortunately it is not. As with nonradicular low back pain, a variety of theories have failed to conclusively identify the exact physiologic or anatomic etiologic abnormality. Such diverse theories as direct neural compression, inflammatory response, biochemical abnormalities, and vascular compromise have yet to explain conclusively the true etiology of the sciatic pain.

Obviously, there is a great deal that we do not understand about the anatomic or physiologic basis for low back pain and sciatica. However, we must not be frustrated by our lack of knowledge. Instead, we must use what we have just discussed as the foundation for understanding the normal ana-

A

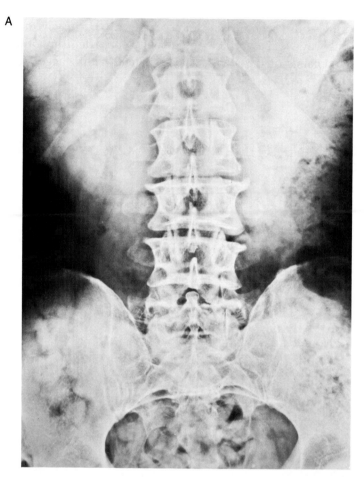

B

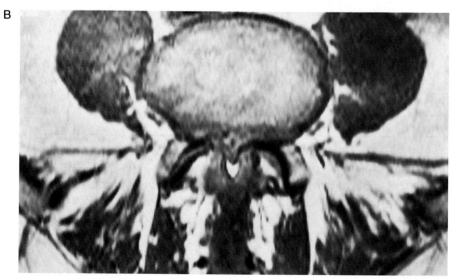

tomic as well as the abnormal anatomic changes occurring in the lumbar spine. In this way we may be able to clinically correlate many of the more common complaints of the low back pain patient with changes seen both anatomically and radiographically.

REFERENCE

1. Nachemson A: The load on lumbar discs in different positions of the body. *Clin Orthop* 1966;45:107–122.

FIG. 2–18. A: Plain radiograph, although not diagnostic, suggests the possibility of spinal stenosis by the abnormally narrowed interlaminar space at L4–5. The subluxation of the facet joints and close approximation of the adjacent spinous processes are characteristic of segmental motion segment degeneration and collapse. **B:** Subluxation of the facet joints, buckling inward of the ligamentum flavum, anterior disc bulging, and arthritic spurring combine to cause signficant spinal stenosis, the endstage of degenerative motion segment collapse.

3

History

"If all else fails, talk to the patient." Probably in no other illness is this statement more appropriate than for the patient with low back pain. In spite of our ability to evaluate the anatomic appearance and function of the lumbar spine with a growing number of diagnostic studies, a few minutes of basic history-taking often affords us more definitive information than thousands of dollars worth of diagnostic tests. In contrast to their success in diagnosing many of the more common ailments affecting the vast majority of the adult population, radiographic and diagnostic studies are often nonproductive in the patient with low back pain. Therefore, it is extremely important that a thorough history be taken of each patient. This will enable the examining physician to order the appropriate diagnostic studies and to avoid unnecessary or delayed treatment.

Although no two patients ever present with the exact same symptom complex, a methodical approach to the history will save time. In addition, an objective approach will help the physician eliminate much of the subjective nature of the patient's complaints and focus only on the objective complaints. This is often difficult with low back pain patients because the primary complaint is most often pain. Unfortunately there is no reliable, reproducible or accurate way to measure pain as if it were a laboratory study or radiograph. Each patient's response to pain is individual. The subjective complaint of pain itself is often not very helpful in arriving at a diagnosis. Thus, a systematic approach to history-taking will enable the physician to sidestep time-consuming dissertations concerning the patients' inability to tolerate their low back pain.

When interviewing a patient, it is important to determine whether the patient has only low back pain *or* low back pain and sciatica. This differentiation has tremendous impact on any subsequent diagnostic studies performed if the patient's symptoms do not improve. For diagnostic simplicity, it is easiest to evaluate first the symptoms related to the low back, then the sciatic or radicular symptoms, and finally the interdependence of the two.

Initial questioning should focus on the onset of the pain. It is important to note the date on which the pain began and whether it was precipitated by a traumatic episode. If the pain began insidiously, a rough approximation of

of pain is important. Patients who relate a specific traumatic event
[on]set of pain should be given an opportunity to explain the nature of
[trau]ma. In the case of an automobile accident, for example, the amount
[of dam]age done to the automobile in which the patient was riding at the time
of the injury may give some insight into the severity of the trauma sustained.
If the patient has been involved in a fall or has suffered direct trauma to the
lumbar spine, the exact anatomic location of the blow or fall should be
described. This information may be helpful when correlating the patient's
current symptoms with those that the physician might expect to follow that
particular type of trauma.

After establishing the onset of the current symptoms, it is important to
determine whether this is the first episode of low back pain. It is also important to determine whether this episode is more or less severe than previous
episodes and whether it has lasted as long as previous episodes. It is also
important to note whether the current level of pain has worsened, improved,
or is unchanged since the initial onset.

Particular attention should be paid to the dynamics of the pain. Specific
questions should be directed at which activities increase or decrease the
pain, especially the activities of walking, standing, sitting, or lying down,
because specific structural abnormalities, such as spinal stenosis or a herniated lumbar disc, are typified by specific pain-related activities.

If there does not appear to be any correlation of the pain with the above
activities, further questioning should be directed at the relationship of the
pain and positional changes such as getting in and out of a chair or bending
forward and straightening up.

Any concomitant stiffness or associated joint complaints are important.
So is the daily pattern of the pain. Early morning stiffness and other joint
complaints raise the possibility of a systemic, rheumatologic, or arthritic
etiology. On the other hand pain in the lumbar spine that is constant, unre-
lated to activity, and awakens the patient from sleep is suggestive of a malignant or metastatic spinal lesion.

The most critical part of the history is to determine whether sciatic pain is
present along with the low back pain. This is extremely important since
almost 90% of patients with low back pain do not have accompanying sciatic pain.

Sciatica derives its name from the sciatic nerve. Therefore true sciatic
pain must follow the anatomic path of the sciatic nerve. The anatomic distribution of the pain allows for the critically important differentiation between
real sciatic pain and referred pain. Authentic sciatic pain must radiate below
the knee and follow one or more of the individual nerve roots that comprise
the sciatic nerve.

In contrast, referred pain may radiate into the hip, buttock, thigh, groin,
and, on occasion, as far distally as the knee. Unfortunately very little is

known about the exact etiology and physiology of referred low back pain. Experimental injections of saline into a variety of the soft tissue supporting structures of the lumbar spine, including the paraspinal muscles, interspinous ligaments, and facet joints produce referred pain in the anatomic areas described above. Although the true etiology of the referred pain pattern is unknown, it is of the utmost importance that it be differentiated from true sciatic pain, which must radiate in the typical dermatomal distribution of the sciatic nerve components.

As with low back pain, the time of onset and progressivity of the sciatic pain should be documented. Patients with sciatica may not have significant (or any) low back pain. The presence of low back pain is important when describing the nature of the sciatic pain. When questioning the patient about the anatomic location of the pain, it is important to know whether there is any associated numbness or weakness in the same anatomic distribution.

Involvement of the L4 nerve root presents with pain radiating into the anterior thigh and medial knee region. L5 nerve root symptoms present with pain over the lateral calf as well as the dorsum of the foot in the first dorsal web space. S1 nerve root pain is most often found over the lateral aspect of the foot.

Just as referred pain must be differentiated from true sciatic pain, so must exaggerated and non-anatomic complaints of neurologic involvement be likewise differentiated. Specific nerve root compression in the lumbar spine does not lead to a "stocking-glove" sensory loss. Complaints of numbness and paresthesias of the entire foot, calf, or lower leg should be viewed with some skepticism and other etiologic causes suspected. Similarly, a patient complaining of recurrent episodes of a leg "giving way" and the patient's falling should also be questioned further. Although lesions involving the actual spinal cord may result in a spastic and awkward gait, it is unusual even for those patients to present with complaints of their legs giving way and their falling. Even if the L5 or S1 nerve root is completely transected, it is more likely that the patient will have a mildly abnormal gait, rather than enough motor loss to lose control of the entire leg and fall, since only very discreet muscular functions are affected.

It is often helpful to include a simple pain drawing for the patient to fill out prior to being seen by the physician. The anatomic distribution of the pain and sensory abnormalities can then be easily observed at the time of the interview. This provides very objective information and usually gives the physician insight into whether the patient's symptoms follow an anatomic distribution (Fig. 3–1). For those patients without the typical dermatomal distribution, additional questioning by the physician is often necessary to differentiate true sciatic pain from pain of a functional or non-neurologic origin.

Patients with neurologic compression in the lumbar spine from any num-

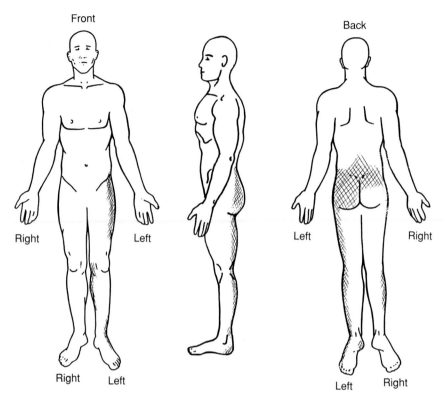

FIG. 3–1. The patient's documentation of painful symptoms on a pain drawing may give meaningful insight into the objectivity of the patient's complaints.

ber of etiologies may rarely present with cauda equina syndrome. The presenting symptoms typically involve bladder and/or bowel dysfunction. These patients may present with or without back and sciatic pain. The neurologic deficits are due to compression of the sacral roots of the cauda equina. Initial urinary symptoms may present as either retention or incontinence. Since compression of the cauda equina results in flaccid paralysis of the bladder, patients may first complain only of retention. Once the bladder fills to capacity, patients will then experience overflow incontinence with frequent small-volume urination.

Cauda equina syndrome, as well as any progressive neurologic deficit of the lower extremities, is the only surgical emergency involving the lumbar spine. Once the cauda equina syndrome is diagnosed clinically or even suspected based on the history and physical examination, prompt diagnostic testing is necessary to avoid needless delay of appropriate and timely treatment.

As with any medical history, the state of the patient's general health should not be overlooked. Any history of malignancy is extremely important in order to assess the possibility of metastatic disease that is often found in the lumbar spine. Recent weight loss, fatigue, change in bowel habits, rectal bleeding, and pulmonary complaints should be investigated. A history of recent febrile episodes or a history of an infectious process may be the cause of low back pain presenting as either an intervertebral disc space infection or vertebral osteomyelitis.

Any systemic disease affecting the patient's endocrine function may have an impact on the patient's low back pain. Almost any endocrine abnormality may have either a direct or indirect effect on calcium metabolism and subsequent osteoporosis or osteopenia. Although the osteopenia itself is not painful, the resultant microfractures and deformities are.

Any history of psychiatric illness may pose difficulties in obtaining an accurate history from the patient. Likewise it is important to ascertain any prescription or illicit drug abuse. It is important not only to know which medications the patients have been taking, but also the quantities and the length of time the patients have been using the drugs. A recent change in the patient's social or economic status may also have an impact on the patient's symptoms. Any unusual stress, such as loss of a job, divorce, or death in the family, may markedly affect the patient's symptom complaints.

Last but not least is the presence of any ongoing litigation or worker's compensation claims, Whether the patient has acquired the services of an attorney, the size of the claim and the length of the time since initiation of the claim are factors that unfortunately may play a significant role in the history and ultimate outcome of the patient's symptoms.

4

Physical Examination

Once a thorough history is taken, it is time for the examining physician to confirm or repudiate his or her clinical impressions by substantiation with the corresponding physical findings. Unfortunately, many of the patients with low back pain without radicular pain may have very few, if any, distinctive physical findings to help in arriving at an appropriate diagnosis. However, the absence of any demonstrable physical abnormalities should not frustrate the examiner but should be used merely as information to confirm that the patient is not having a more significant or complicated spinal problem. On the other hand, patients who have a relatively unremarkable history must still have a thorough physical examination to insure that, despite a lackluster history, they do not have a more serious problem.

The physical examination should begin with a general inspection of the spine in the standing position. No patient can be adequately examined while wearing clothes. All patients should be examined with their gown opened posteriorly. This facilitates easy inspection of the spine as well as easy access to direct palpation.

An inspection of the spine from behind the patient should reveal no asymmetry of the ribs, flank, or pelvis. Likewise the head should be directly aligned over the middle of the sacrum. Any deviation from this perfectly symmetrical appearance may be due to a scoliotic or lateral deformity of the spine (Fig. 4–1).

The spine is not straight in the anteroposterior plane but has normal anatomic curvatures. The patient should be examined from the side to best visualize the normal sagittal curvatures (Fig. 4–2). The normal cervical lordosis, thoracic kyphosis, and lumbar lordosis should maintain proper balance of the head and trunk over the pelvic girdle. Any increase or decrease in these normal curvatures should be noted. After inspection of spinal alignment, the skin of the trunk and pelvis should be inspected for the presence of any congenital abnormalities. Any hairy patch, areas of pigmentation, skin dimpling, or lipomatous masses should be noted. Obviously any healed surgical scars should be documented with particular attention to the exact anatomic location of the scar.

Following this general inspection, it is time to examine the spine directly.

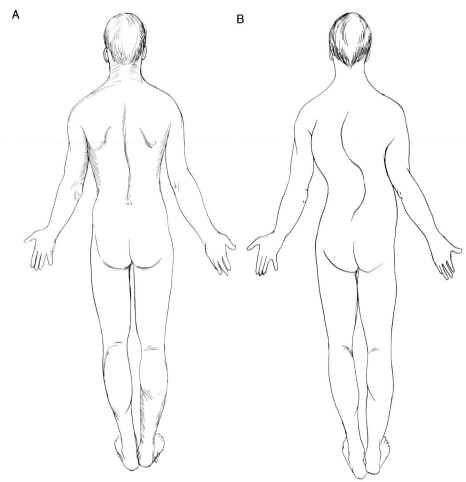

FIG. 4–1. A: The patient's spine should be examined in the standing position. There should be no asymmetry of the hips, pelvis, or flanks. The skin
of the trunk should be examined in search of any cutaneous lesions suggestive of an intraspinal congenial abnormality. **B:** Asymmetry of the flank
or lateral list of the trunk is often caused by a lumbar scoliosis. Radiographs
are necessary to determine whether the curvature is due to a true structural
abnormality or a functional curvature secondary to a painful spinal disorder.

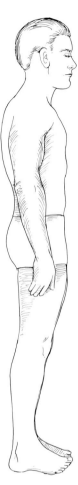

FIG. 4–2. The normal cervical lordosis, thoracic kyphosis, and lumbar lordosis should be evident when viewing the patient from the side. Any loss of these normal curvatures should be noted.

The midline should be palpated first by feeling for the spinous process and then moving inferiorly to the interspace until the next spinous process is palpated. This technique should begin in the thoracic region and continue distally to the lumbosacral junction. This systematic approach will enable the examiner to locate a discretely painful anatomic location. If performed carefully, the examiner may be able to differentiate bony pain at the spinous process from ligamentous pain in the interspace. In addition to eliciting any painful areas, this orderly approach is an excellent way to assess the normal spinal alignment. Any loss or increase in the normal lumbar lordosis is easily palpable even in the most obese patients. Most spondylolisthesis (proba-

bly the most common segmental abnormality of alignment of the lumbosacral spine) may be palpated by feeling for the step-off between the two
adjacent spinous processes (Fig. 4–3).

Palpation of the posterior iliac spine should be done to insure that the
pelvis is level and that no pelvic obliquity is present. If pelvic obliquity is
present, it should be determined whether the obliquity is due to a leg length
discrepancy or an intrinsic pelvic abnormality by further diagnostic testing.

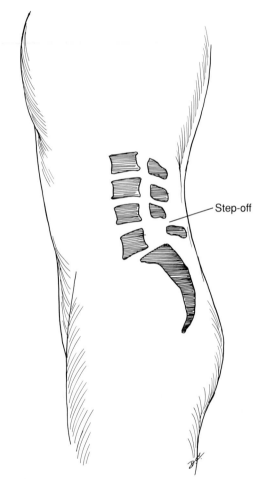

FIG. 4–3. Spondylolisthesis may frequently be missed on visual inspection
but often diagnosed by serial palpation of the spinous processes. Depending on the type of spondylolisthesis, the palpable step-off may be felt at the
level of the slip (degenerative spondylolisthesis) or at the level just above
the slip (lytic spondylolisthesis).

After palpation of the midline, the paraspinal muscles should be examined. Any painful areas, particularly those with asymmetric muscular tone, should be noted as to their anatomic location. Asymmetric tightness or muscle spasm may result in the patient's listing to one side, thus producing "sciatic" scoliosis. This is a nonstructural deformity and will correct itself once the painful stimuli is removed.

Painful, circumscribed areas of muscular tenderness are often referred to as trigger points. Although there has been a wide variety of treatment modalities proposed to alleviate this type of pain, the exact etiology or underlying pathology for these localized painful muscular areas is not known. Frequently, subcutaneous, well-circumscribed lipomatous masses are found overlying and adjacent to the posterior iliac crest. Although these small masses may often become painful, the cause of the pain is not understood.

Any midline or paraspinal areas of discomfort should also be percussed. Pain with percussion is frequently seen in patients with infectious processes involving the spine or its adjacent structures.

While the patient is still standing, the range of motion should be assessed. With the knees maintained in the fully extended position, forward flexion is measured by the distance from the finger tips to the floor. This allows reproducible measurements for comparison with the patient acting as his own baseline control. Extension is somewhat harder to measure objectively, but, with the patient standing, the lumbar spine is extended posteriorly and measured in degrees of change from the normal upright position. Similar angular measurements are made for right and left lateral bending as well as rotation of the lumbar spine. Any precipitated pain down the leg should be noted during the specific maneuver performed by the patient.

Following examination of spinal alignment, trunk musculature, and flexibility, a thorough neurologic examination must be performed. While still in the standing position, the patient's gait should be observed to assess any obvious abnormalities in normal gait pattern. A variety of gait abnormalities such as spasticity, dropfoot, and ataxia may provide vital information as to the etiologic abnormalities responsible for the abnormal gait pattern.

Prior to manually testing motor strength, the patient should attempt both heel walking and toe walking. An alternative to this portion of the exam may be repetitive heel and toe elevation on one foot while balancing or holding onto the sink or examination table (Fig. 4–4). This may actually allow the examiner to observe more discrete motor asymmetry than with heel and toe walking. Heel elevation is principally a measure of S1 nerve root innervation of the gastrocsoleus group. Any asymmetry of repetitive toe elevation may be caused by weakness of either the L4 innervated anterior tibialis and/ or the L5 innervated extensor hallucis longus.

Manual motor testing is best performed with the patient in a sitting posi-

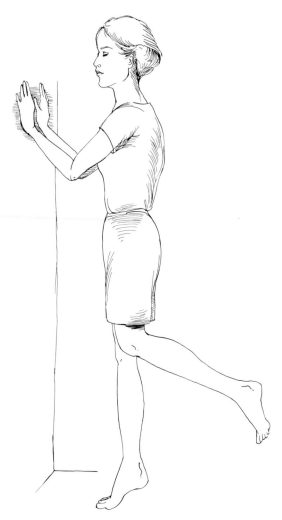

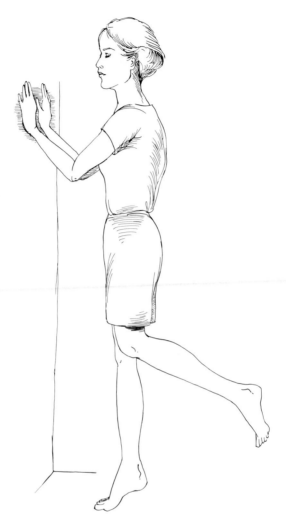

FIG. 4–4. Repetitive heel and toe elevation may reveal more subtle neurologic asymmetry than is evident with heel and toe walking. Repetitive testing may also reveal evidence of asymmetric fatigue not usually apparent with manual motor testing.

tion with the legs hanging freely over the edge of the examining table (Table 4–1). Motor testing is best measured on the traditional 0–5 scale. This type of objective rating system allows for reproducible and comparative examinations to be done in the future with more clinical objectivity.

Hip flexion is performed principally by the iliopsoas muscle, which is innervated by the T12, L1, L2, and L3 nerve roots. The quadriceps muscle allowing thigh extension is innervated by the L2, L3, and L4 branches of the femoral nerve. The hip adductor muscles are innerverted by the L2, L3, and

TABLE 4–1. Lower extremity motor testing

Nerve Root Level	Muscle
T12, L1, L2, L3	Iliopsoas
L2, L3, L4	Quadriceps
	Hip adductor
L4	Tibialis anterior
L5	Extensor hallucis longus
	Gluteus medius
	Extensor Digitorum longus, brevis
S1	Gastrocsoleus
	Peroneus longus, brevis
	Gluteus maximus

L4 branches of the obturator nerve. The function of the L4 nerve root is best evaluated by testing the strength of the tibialis anterior muscle, which allows for dorsiflexion and inversion of the foot.

Function of the L5 nerve root is best demonstrated by testing the strength of the extensor hallucis longus. Resistance to great toe extension during the examination should be across the metatarsophalangeal joint and not the interphalangeal joint. This provides easier assessment of strength than at the weaker and less stable interphalangeal joint. Another measure of L5 root function, although somewhat less sensitive, is the gluteus medius strength and the long and short toe extensors.

The function of the S1 nerve root is most easily evaluated by testing the strength of the gastrocsoleus or plantar flexion. Additional measures of S1 function are the gluteus maximus, peroneus longus, and peroneus brevis muscles. The S2, S3, and S4 nerve roots supply the intrinsic muscles of the foot. Any deformity of the forefoot or toes should raise the possibility of a neurologic etiology.

Sensation of the lower extremities should be assessed by checking both pin or deep pain sensation, as well as light touch sensation (Fig 4–5). The L1, L2, and L3 nerve roots provide sensation over the anterior thigh. The sensory distribution of the L4 nerve root is over the medial aspect of the leg and demarcated from the sensory supply of the L5 nerve root by the anterior crest of the tibia. Sensation over the lateral leg and dorsum of the foot particularly in the first dorsal web space is supplied by the L5 nerve root. The S1 nerve root provides sensation over the lateral and plantar aspects of the foot. Perianal sensation is supplied by the S2, S3, S4, and S5 nerve roots in a concentric manner. The outermost ring is innervated by the S2 nerve root, while the innermost area is supplied by the S4 and S5 roots.

The reflex examination should be done not only to ascertain the absence of a normal reflex but also to delineate any asymmetry between the right and left sides. The knee jerk or patellar reflex is tested to determine L4 nerve

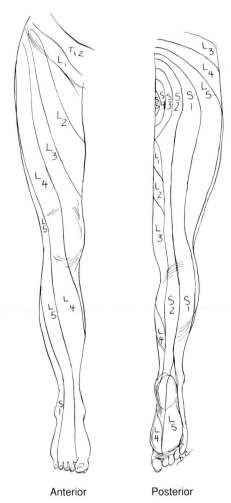

Anterior   Posterior

FIG. 4–5. Abnormal sensory loss should follow the anatomic dermatomes outlined above. "Stocking glove" or nondermatomal loss should alert the examiner to a pathologic process other than discrete nerve root compression.

root dysfunction. Unfortunately, the innervation is not solely from the L4 nerve root, but there are also contributions from the L2 and L3 nerve roots, although significantly less than the L4 nerve root. The tibialis posterior reflex is a measure of L5 nerve root function but is not easily reproducible and frequently not as satisfactory a diagnostic test as either the knee or ankle reflex. Alteration of the ankle jerk reflects S1 nerve root abnormalities. The superficial anal reflex may be tested by stimulating the perianal skin and observing for anal sphincter contraction. This reflex is supplied by the S2, S3, and S4 nerve roots.

The presence of hyper-reflexia and, more important, unsustained or sustained clonus while testing the knee or ankle reflex is indicative of an upper motor neuron lesion. The same holds true for the presence of a Babinski or Oppenheim response. Any of these abnormal reflex changes should lead to further investigation of a possible pathologic lesion proximal to the lumbar spine at either the spinal cord or brain level.

Proprioception should be checked by simple flexion and extension of the great toe and ankle. Although altered proprioception is rarely a predominant symptom in lumbar spine abnormalities, it may result from a neurologic abnormality proximal to the cauda equina at the spinal cord and/or brain level/or a systemic metabolic disease such as diabetes.

At the conclusion of the peripheral neurologic examination, the presence of pulses in both feet should be verified. It is often difficult to differentiate the radicular pain of arterial insufficiency from spinal stenosis in the elderly patient. The absence of pulses in a symptomatic patient necessitates further peripheral vascular evaluation prior to an expensive radiographic evaluation of the lumbar spine.

Any tests or maneuvers that elicit or recreate the patient's pain or symptoms should be done at the conclusion of the examination. This is done mainly to avoid aggravating the patient's pain and allowing full cooperation in the earlier portion of the physical examination. These maneuvers are done principally to evaluate the presence of any neural irritability. Neural irritability typically results in sciatic pain radiating down the affected extremity in the same anatomic distribution experienced by the patient. As with true sciatic pain, it must follow the distribution of one or more of the sciatic nerve components radiating below the knee, unless the pain arises from involvement of any of the femoral nerve components. In these patients the radicular pain is found in the anterior thigh.

The most common and probably most misunderstood test for neural irritability is the straight leg raising test. Straight leg raising may be done with the patient either in the sitting or lying position (Fig. 4–6.) While the patient is in the lying position, the examiner should grasp the patient's heel and raise the entire lower extremity with the knee fully extended. The angle of elevation from the horizontal at which the patient begins to experience true sciatic or radicular pain is a positive straight leg raising test. Pain elicited only in the low back or buttocks is not a positive straight leg raising test since no sciatic pain is provoked. It is important to differentiate a truly positive straight leg raising test from hamstring tightness. It is quite common to produce posterior thigh pain when tightness of the hamstring muscles is present. Once again, true sciatic pain must be produced to have a positive straight leg raising test and must be differentiated from referred or hamstring pain.

A

B

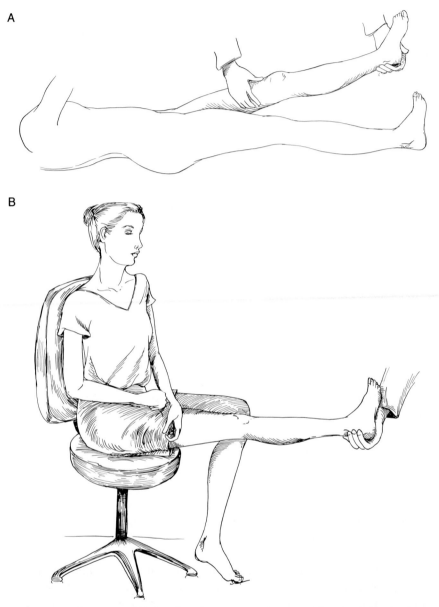

FIG. 4–6. The straight leg raising test may be done in the sitting or lying position. **A:** In the lying position elevation of the lower extremity must produce sciatic pain to be considered a positive straight leg raising test. No matter how painful the provoked back or hamstring pain, only provocation of true sciatic pain should be considered a positive straight leg raising test. **B:** When the straight leg raising test is performed in the sitting position, the hips must remain flexed 90° with the trunk maintained perpendicular to the floor in order to insure an accurate response.

The straight leg raising test may be performed in the sitting position. The patient should have the hips and knees flexed at 90 degrees while the examiner grasps the heel and elevates the leg slowly to full extension of the knee. The angle of elevation should be noted at the time at which the patient begins to experience sciatic pain. If the straight leg raising test is negative in the supine or sitting position, passive dorsiflexion of the ankle may elicit neural irritability once the leg has been fully extended.

Normally the asymptomatic or contralateral lower extremity should not elicit sciatic pain when performing the straight leg raising test. However, if straight leg raising of the asymptomatic leg produces sciatic pain radiating down the opposite or symptomatic leg, this is strong evidence of neural irritability. This finding is known as the positive contralateral straight leg raising test.

Another reliable test of neural irritability is the bowstring test. This is performed while the patient is in either the supine or sitting position. If in the supine position, a straight leg raising maneuver is performed until sciatic pain is produced. Following pain production, the knee is flexed 15–20 degrees until the pain is relieved. The examiner then uses his free hand to palpate the tibial nerve in the popliteal fossa. Normally no pain is produced unless one or more of the component nerve roots is affected. A positive response will produce pain radiating proximally or distal to the knee joint and is often accompanied by paresthesias. This is a very sensitive test for neural irritability and is probably more reliable than the straight leg raising maneuver.

The bowstring test may also be performed while the patient is in the sitting position, much like the sitting straight leg raising test. Once the foot is elevated to the position that produces sciatic pain, the foot is lowered 10–15 degrees, and the popliteal fosa is palpated with the free hand. Production of radicular pain signifies a positive test.

Involvement of any of the components of the femoral nerve do not typically present with positive findings with any of the above sciatic nerve stretch tests. This is primarily due to its more anterior exit from the pelvis. The best test for femoral nerve irritability is the reverse straight leg raising test. This is performed with the patient in the prone position and the lower extremity passively extended at the hip. Pain radiating into the anterior thigh is considered a positive reverse straight leg raising test consistent with femoral nerve irritability.

It is not uncommon for patients with low back disorders to complain about "sacroiliac" pain. However, it is quite unusual for a patient to have symptoms emanating from the sacroiliac articulation unless there is involvement of the sacroiliac joint with infection, significant trauma, or spondyloarthritis. Despite the infrequent occurrence of true sacroiliac pain, it is easily examined by several maneuvers designed to elicit pain with motion of the sacroiliac joint.

While the patient is in the supine position, the examiner places one hand on each iliac crest and the pelvis compressed toward the midline. Pain elicited with this maneuver suggests an abnormality of the sacroiliac joint.

Gaenslen's sign is seen when pain is provoked by extending the patient's lower extremity over the side of the examining table with the opposite leg flexed at the hip and knee. Pain present in the area of the sacroiliac joint is indicative of abnormal sacroiliac joint function.

While examining the sacroiliac joint, it is also important to examine the hip joint. Intra-articular hip disease may often radiate into the groin, buttocks, and as far distally as the knee. Although hip disease is usually distinguishable from the symptoms of spinal stenosis, the two pathologic conditions may co-exist. Therefore, it is important to determine which pathologic condition is contributing the most significant portion of the patient's symptoms. This can be easily evaluated by passively ranging the patient's hips and observing whether the pain elicited recreates the patient's symptoms. Earlier in the examination, any abductor lurch consistent with primary hip disease should also have been evident.

Once the examination has ended, a truly objective record of any positive neurologic or mechanical findings will be clear. In addition to any abnormal objective findings demonstrated during the examination, it is also helpful to simply observe how the patient sits, changes position, and generally moves about. A great deal of understanding of how well the patient is able to cope with the pain as well as any exaggerated response to any portions of the examination will be evident. This gives the physician additional insight into the overall character of the patient, which may be critical when it comes time to begin diagnostic testing and formulating therapeutic plans.

5

Radiographic and Laboratory Tests

Physicians who treat radiographs rather than patients will soon realize that their clinical success rate is rather disappointing. Ordering or reviewing radiographic studies should not be done until the history and physical examination are completed. This will not only save the patient money by not undergoing unnecessary studies, but will also prevent the physician's becoming clinically biased by focusing on a radiographic abnormality that may have no bearing on the patient's symptoms. Many of the findings on plain radiographs, CT scans, MRI, and myelography have little clinical relevance unless they correlate exactly with the patient's clinical history and physical findings. It cannot be emphasized enough that these ancillary studies should be used only to confirm or rule out a potential abnormality suspected solely on the patient's presumptive diagnosis arrived at directly from the history and physical examination. In other words, "if all else fails, examine the patient." If one follows this simple rule, a large number of unnecessary and superfluous studies will be avoided without the economic cost and frustration for the patient.

Plain radiographs of the lumbosacral spine are probably the most overused study of all those available in the diagnostic armamentarium for lumbar spine disease. The cost-effectiveness of plain radiographs of the lumbar spine is very low since their correlation with the patient's symptoms is quite poor. It is more likely that the degenerative abnormalities noted on the spinal radiographs, particularly in older patients, are only radiographic documentation of the normal aging process.

There is wide agreement that the degenerative changes of the lumbar spine seen on radiographs have no consistent correlation to the patient's symptoms. Only one study of 321 patients found any correlation between patients' symptoms and radiographic findings (5). The two significant radiographic abnormalities were the presence of disc narrowing and traction spurs at the L4–5 level only. The patients with these findings tended to have a higher incidence of severe low back pain than patients with more normal

radiographs. There was also a higher incidence of extremity pain and neurologic loss when these two abnormalities were present at the L4–5 level.

However, before accepting these findings as truly clinically significant,
one needs to look only at several other large studies that found none of these
same correlations. One large study examining the radiographs of 238 back
pain patients with low back pain and sciatica as well as radiographs from 66
normal patients found no such correlation (13). In contrast to the previous
study, there was no increased incidence of low back pain or sciatica with the
radiographic presence of disc degeneration or spondylosis (Fig. 5–1). Similar frustrating results have been reported with other studies that attempt to

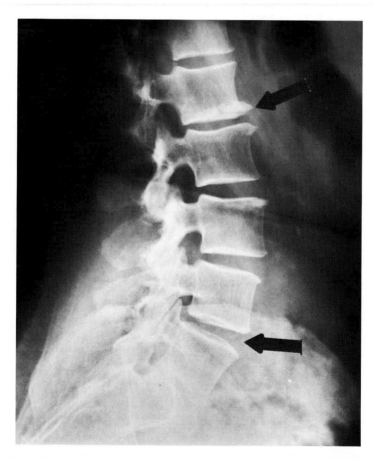

FIG. 5–1. Despite these rather ominous radiographic abnormalities such
as the disc space narrowing (*arrow*) and osteophyte formation, there is no
clinical correlation of these findings with attempts to explain the painful
symptoms.

correlate the presence of degenerative radiographic abnormalities with the clinical symptomatology.

Thus it appears that plain radiographs have very little diagnostic value for the average patient with low back pain. The presence of transitional vertebrae, vacuum disc signs, disc space narrowing, claw spurs, spondylosis, and Schmorl's nodes have no documented correlation with an increased incidence and severity of low back pain (Fig. 5–2).

Those patients for whom no clearcut diagnosis can be made based on the history and the physical examination but who have any number of the above abnormalities present on their plain radiographs, the physician is tempted to

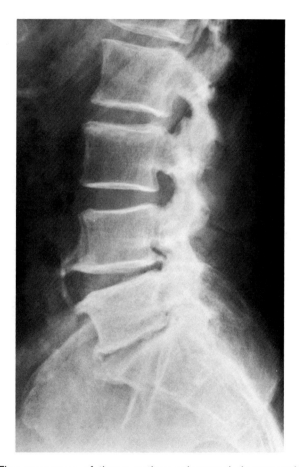

FIG. 5–2. The presence of these rather advanced degenerative changes have no correlation with the incidence or severity of low back pain. It is more likely that they are only radiographic evidence of the normal aging process.

label as having degenerative spine disease or arthritis of the spine. Once identified as having symptoms secondary to a "degenerative" or "arthritic" spine, it is then quite easy for the physician to prescribe any number of the arthritic or anti-inflammatory medications. However, the physician must realize that almost 70% of all adult lumbar spine films will demonstrate radiographic evidence of degenerative disease. Common sense dictates that all of these patients do not need to be taking medication prescribed solely on the appearance of the radiographs that do not correlate with any of the patient's symptoms (Fig. 5–3).

In general, lumbosacral radiographs should not be a routine part of the initial evaluation of the patient with low back pain. However, that does not mean that this basic radiographic study should never be ordered. To the contrary, any patient with a history and/or physical examination suggesting a neoplastic, infectious, traumatic, metabolic, or structural abnormality should have these radiographs performed as part of the initial examination (Fig. 5–4). There is no excuse for not obtaining plain radiographs when a patient complains of atypical, unremitting pain that may be caused by a primary or metastatic lesion of the lumbar spine. Any patient, particularly an elderly patient, with a history of cancer or with persistent or increasing low back pain with or without sciatica should have lumbosacral radiographs to rule out the presence of a primary or metastatic tumor (Fig. 5–5).

The same guidelines hold true for any patient with a long history suggesting a systemic, infectious, or metabolic disease that may affect the spine. Patients will readily accept what may appear to be an unnecessary radiograph if the physician explains the clinical concerns and why the study is being ordered. It is far easier to explain this to an anxious patient than explaining a tumor or infectious lesion discovered after months of clinical neglect. The best rule of thumb is to order the lumbosacral radiographs any time there is even the slightest indication that a significant structural abnormality may be present. Fortunately for the patient and physician, the number of patients presenting with these clinical signs and symptoms are in the minority.

In patients with neurologic symptoms, plain radiographs are not particularly helpful when attempting to identify neural compression. Unless there is a destructive bony lesion, a significant deformity or spondylolisthesis present, plain radiographs will not be helpful in arriving at a diagnosis. Remember, plain radiographs show details of the bony anatomy only. In patients with neurologic signs and symptoms, it is the visualization of the soft tissues, particularly of the neural elements, that will allow a definitive diagnosis.

The presence of degenerative disc disease and disc space narrowing should not be confused with a herniated disc—clinically or radiographically

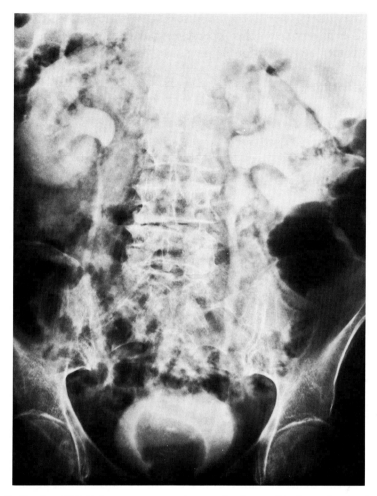

FIG. 5–3. An IVP (intravenous pyelogram) of an elderly patient who had never had an episode of low back pain in his life. Although it is tempting to treat radiographs such as these, the physician must always remember to "treat patients, not x-rays."

(Fig. 5–6). Unfortunately, many patients as well as physicians consider degenerative disc disease and disc herniation one and the same despite their distinctly different pathophysiologic etiologies.

In years past, the radiographic diagnosis of any type of intraspinal neural compression was often difficult and nondiagnostic. Oil-based intrathecal contrast agents such as Pantopaque left a great deal to be desired as a diagnostic tool. Aside from the significant morbidity associated with its use, including post-myelogram reactions and arachnoiditis, the radiographic im-

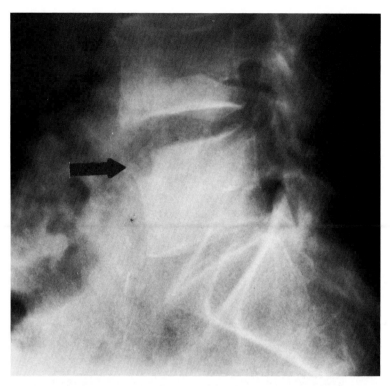

FIG. 5–4. Routine lateral radiograph of a 38-year-old male complaining of unremitting pain not relieved with rest. Closed needle biopsy revealed a staphlococous osteomyelitis involving the anterior vertebral body of L5 (*arrow*).

ages of the neural elements, particularly the individual nerve roots, were often difficult to visualize.

Fortunately, the oil-based contrast agents are no longer being used since the introduction of water soluble contrast agents such as metrizamide and iohexol. These agents allow for markedly improved visualization of the thoracic spinal cord, the conus medullaris, and the individual nerve roots exiting the neural foramen. With better visualization of the intrathecal contents and the significantly lower morbidity associated with their use, the water soluble agents have replaced the oil-based contrast agents as diagnostic tools in the radiographic analysis of the patient with neurologic symptoms (Fig. 5–7).

As the use of water soluble myeolography became widespread, computerized axial tomography of the lumbosacral spine was also gaining popularity. Transverse images as well as coronal and sagittal reconstructions added a new dimension to the radiographic evaluation of the lumbar spine. With the

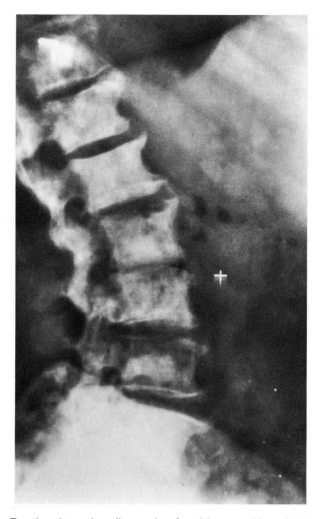

FIG. 5–5. Routine lateral radiograph of a 63-year-old male treated three years previously for cancer of the prostate. Progressive back pain led to the radiographic diagnosis of disseminated metastatic disease of the thoracolumbar spine.

ability to view the spinal anatomy from this new perspective, the diagnosis of a number of intraspinal abnormalities was simplified. The ability to visualize the neural elements was further enhanced with the addition of intravenous contrast or following the intrathecal injection of contrast after myelography (Fig. 5–8).

Despite these tremendous advances over oil-based myelography, both water soluble myelography and CT scans have their limitations. Water soluble myelography is still an invasive procedure. Although the morbidity

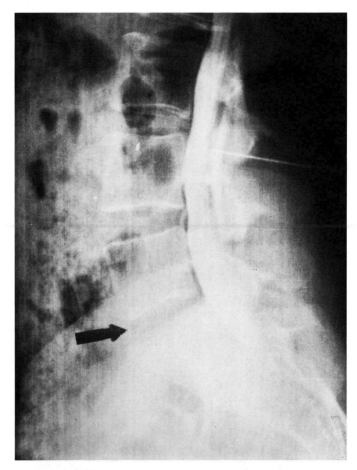

FIG. 5–6. Degenerative disc disease and a herniated lumbar disc should never be confused. The degenerative disc narrowing at L5-S1 (*arrow*), should not be mistaken for a herniated disc. Note there is absolutely no distortion of the contrast at this level that would be characteristic of a herniated lumbar disc.

associated with its use is low and often short-lived, there persists a small group of patients who experience post-myelogram headaches, urinary retention, and a variety of temporary but worrisome central nervous system reactions. It is interesting that, in one study examining the incidence of post-myelogram reactions, the number of patients experiencing adverse reactions was significantly higher in those having normal myelograms than in those with abnormal findings (6). The outcome of this study reiterates the fact that myelography is truly an invasive procedure and should be reserved for those patients thought to have true neurologic compression based on their

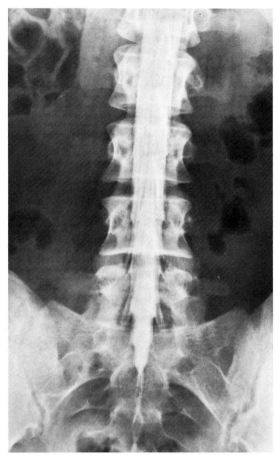

FIG. 5–7. Normal water soluble myelogram. Note the excellent depiction of the individual neural elements throughout the lumbar spine. This detail was not previously available with oil-based contrast agents.

clinical signs and symptoms. Myelography should never be used as a screening tool.

Another limitation of myelography is its inability to visualize the neurologic elements distal to a complete block of the contrast agent (Fig. 5–9). Thus it is impossible to determine whether there is any concomitant intraspinal pathology distal to the blockage. Post-myelogram CT scanning is particularly helpful in these cases and should always be utilized in the patient with a complete myelographic block.

One of the major limitations of CT scanning is its inability to detect intrathecal lesions adjacent to the anatomic structures scanned. Patients with lesions of the conus or lower thoracic spinal cord may on occasion present

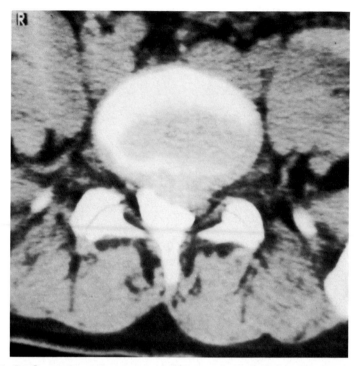

FIG. 5–8. Contrast-enhanced computerized tomography (CT) scan demonstrating a large L5-S1 disc herniation clearly showing the displacement of the nerve root and dural sac.

with clinical symptoms more suggestive of cauda equina compression. A routine lumbar CT scan would not detect these lesions unless the clinical findings were suggestive of a higher anatomic lesion, which may often not be the case.

Even with these drawbacks, myelography and CT scanning have become commonplace as the diagnostic studies utilized in the workup of the patient with neurologic signs and symptoms. As their popularity grew, so did the controversy as to which of these two modalities was best at diagnosing lesions of the lumbar spine.

A number of studies have attempted to resolve this controversy, but unfortunately the conclusions of these studies did not result in a clearcut answer as to which is the best diagnostic study. One large study consisted of 461 patients undergoing CT scans and myelography (11). The results were unable to conclusively predict that one study was diagnostically superior to the other. In patients with a herniated disc, the sensitivity of myelography was 82% compared to 73% with CT scanning. However, the inverse was true for the specificity of myelography at 67% compared to 77% for CT

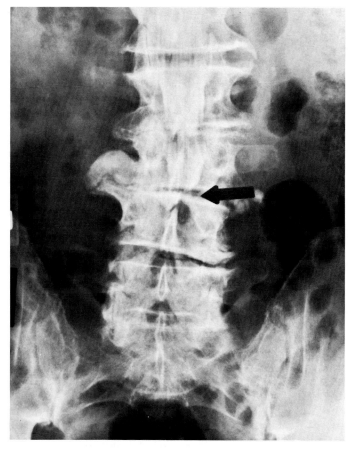

FIG. 5–9. A lumbar myelogram with an incomplete obstruction at L2-3 and a complete block of the contrast agent at L3-4 (*arrow*). Without further radiographic studies, it is impossible to determine the presence of any neurologic compression distal to the obstruction.

scanning. To further confuse the data, the positive predictive value of the two studies showed no statistically significant difference at 93% and 94%.

Another study showed similar insignificant clinical superiority between the two studies when comparing the surgical findings in 134 patients with CT and myelographic abnormalities (4). Myelography correlated in 94% of the cases while CT scanning correlated in 92%. Once again no clearcut difference between the two studies exists.

Despite these ambiguous findings, there have been studies that tend to support the accuracy of myelography over CT scanning. One study examining the surgical findings in 122 patients with either a herniated disc or spinal stenosis found myelography to be more accurate than CT scanning in disc herniations (83% versus 72%) as well as in spinal stenosis (93% versus 89%) (2).

Another study supporting myelography compared the dimensions of the spinal canal on myelography and CT scanning prior to surgical decompression for spinal stenosis. The CT scan dimensions correlated clinically in only 20% of patients compared to an 83% accuracy of the myelographic measurements (3).

Although there appears to be a slight tendency to favor myelography as a diagnostic tool in patients with neurologic findings, this controversy is certainly not resolved. Despite the apparently higher accuracy found with myelography, it must be remembered that myelography is an invasive study with a small but recognized morbidity. In this setting the physician must be faced with the dilemma of subjecting a patient to an invasive procedure or be satisfied with a diagnostic study that may not have quite as good clinical accuracy.

Fortunately this dilemma may be in the process of being resolved as the use of magnetic resonance imaging (MRI) becomes more widespread and technologically advanced. As improvements and innovations in the development of surface coils continue, the use of MRI is rapidly becoming more commonplace than either myelography or CT scanning. MRI has the advantage over both myelography and CT scanning of being totally non-invasive and without the potential risk associated with radiation exposure. It is also much closer to myelography than CT scanning in providing a dynamic and complete study of the spinal contents on the sagittal projection (Fig. 5–10). With improved surface coils, the transverse images are also approaching and, in many cases, surpassing the quality of CT scans.

The MRI also has the ability to determine early degenerative changes occurring in the intervertebral disc not normally detected by myelography or CT scanning (Fig. 5–11). However, one must be wary of this increased sensitivity of the MRI to detect early degenerative changes of the disc and not be tricked into over-diagnosis and treatment. Remember, it is always best to treat patients and not radiographic abnormalities if one is to have a high rate of clinical success.

Early comparative studies are reporting that MRI may be superior to the other diagnostic studies, particularly in the diagnosis of the lumbar disc herniation and intrathecal lesions. One study comparing the accuracy of CT scanning, myelography, CT-myelography and MRI, found MRI to be the most accurate when comparing the diagnostic study to the operative findings in 59 patients. The accuracy of the MRI was 76.5%, slightly better than the myelo-CT (7). The MRI also appears to be somewhat better at diagnosing sequestered disc fragments than the alternative diagnostic studies (Fig. 5–12). The MRI was found to have an 89% sensitivity, 82% specificity, and

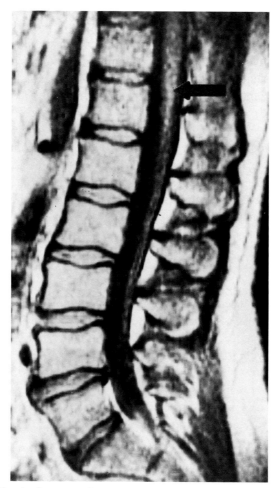

FIG. 5–10. Sagittal magnetic resonance imaging (MRI) demonstrating the distal spinal cord, conus medullarus (*arrow*), and the cauda equina, providing a much more dynamic representation of the neural elements.

an 85% accuracy in distinquishing sequestered disc herniations from other types of herniations based on the operative findings in 20 patients (8).

MRI enhanced with the IV contrast gadolinium has been shown to be extremely helpful in those patients with recurrent symptoms following previous lumbar spine surgery. The gadolinium allows differentiation of postoperative scar formation from the avascular recurrent disc fragment (Fig. 5–13). The ability to differentiate postoperative scar tissue from true mechanical compression of the neural elements with gadolinium enhancement allows for ease of diagnosis not currently available with myelography or even contrast-enhanced CT scanning. For those patients with intrathecal as

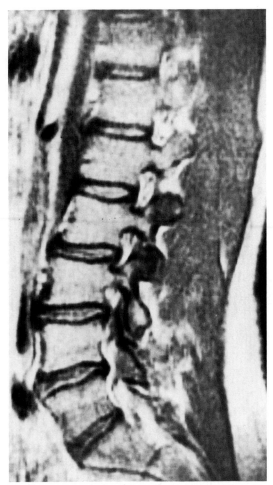

FIG. 5–11. The sensitivity of the MRI at detecting early degenerative changes of the intervertebral disc far exceeds the diagnostic ability of myelography or CT. However, one must be careful to avoid over-diagnosis with this extremely sensitive study.

well as extradural lesions, gadolinium enhancement also provides excellent visualization of the extent of the mass within the spinal canal (Fig. 5–14).

It appears that MRI is rapidly becoming the diagnostic study of choice in many of the lumbar spine abnormalities presenting with neurologic signs and symptoms. This is particularly true in patients with a suspected herniated disc or intrathecal lesion. Perhaps the only area in which MRI has not replaced myelography as the procedure of choice is in patients suspected of having lateral recess or spinal stenosis. With time and improved technological advances it is likely that the ability of the MRI to better visualize the

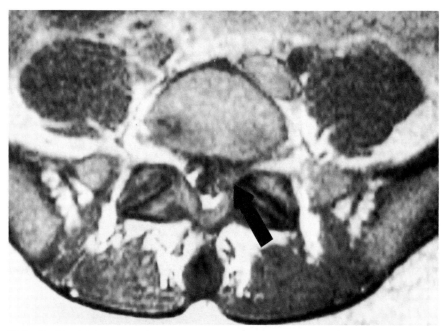

FIG. 5–12. MRI demonstrating a large sequestered L5-S1 disc herniation (*arrow*) obliterating the nerve root and displacing the dural sac.

lateral recesses and the critical spinal canal diameter will surpass the diagnostic capabilities of myelography in the patient with spinal stenosis.

Discography is probably the most controversial of all the diagnostic procedures available for the workup of the patient with lumbar spine disease. For many years, discography has served a two-fold purpose. The first aspect of discography is the radiographic appearance of the contrast-enhanced disc on the plain radiographs (Fig. 5–15). The second aspect is the clinical response of the patient after the injection of contrast. This is commonly known as the provocation test in which the patient's back and sciatic symptoms are attempted to be recreated with the injection of contrast. If the patient reports reproduction of the pain in the usual distribution, the provocation test is reported to be positive.

For many years it was believed that a normal disc would accept only up to 1 cc of contrast at the time of injection or otherwise be classified as degenerative or incompetent. Despite these rather common claims, there is no experimental or clinical data to confirm this.

As the quality of CT scans continued to improve over the years, discography was no longer used solely with plain radiography. The injected disc visualized with CT scanning yielded far better details of the interdiscal pa-

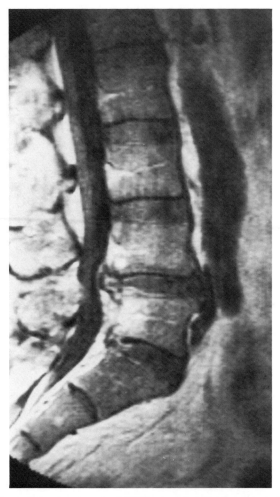

FIG. 5–13. Gadolinium-enhanced MRI showing a recurrent disc herniation at L4-5. Although there is a thin shell of contrast-enhanced epidural scarring overlying the avascular recurrent disc herniation, it is clear that the displacement of the dural sac is due to a recurrent disc herniation and not postoperative scarring.

thology than with plain radiographs (Fig. 5–16). Since CT discography has become routine for those advocates of discography, a number of grading systems have been proposed to quantify the extent of the disc disruption and pathology (10).

A new theory has been proposed to explain the low back pain in patients with longstanding chronic pain that is nonradiating and unassociated with neurologic symptoms. Based on the CT discographic appearance, some advocates of discography have described a pathologic condition known as *in-*

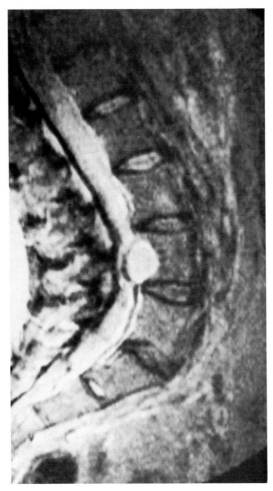

FIG. 5–14. Gadolinium-enhanced MRI illustrating a well-circumscribed mass eroding the vertebral body of L4 and causing extradural compression of the thecal sac.

ternal disc disruption. In those patients whose pain is attributed to internal disc disruption, there is alteration of the normal concentric annular architecture leading to degenerative changes on the CT-discogram and thus the term *internal disc disruption.* It is the internal derangement of the normal disc anatomy and the ensuing degenerative changes that have been proposed as the etiology for the low back pain. Unfortunately, there is wide disagreement on this theory and no scientific data has conclusively proved the correlation between abnormal CT discography and the presence of low back pain.

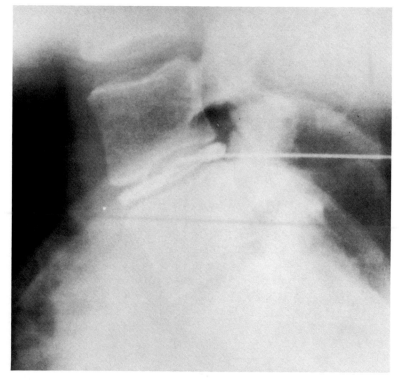

FIG. 5–15. Discogram revealing a degenerative disc with layering of the contrast throughout the extent of the disc.

Despite the lack of universal acceptance of this theory, many physicians will recommend lumbar fusion for patients presenting with internal disc disruption on CT discography. Even in the presence of a positive provocation test and abnormal CT appearance, there is no conclusive data supporting CT discography as the sole diagnostic study for the preoperative workup of the patient suspected of needing a lumbar fusion. Before recommending surgical fusion, it would be prudent to have additional diagnostic criteria to support the recommendation of lumbar fusion.

As with CT scanning itself, CT discography may slowly be replaced by the MRI (12). The ability of the MRI far exceeds the ability of the CT scan to diagnose early degenerative changes within the disc. In fact the MRI is able to depict almost any of the anatomic abnormalities seen on CT discography. The sensitivity of the MRI in visualizing early degenerative changes is so great that, in many cases of early degenerative change, the diagnosis of internal disc derangement may be inappropriate since the suspected pathologic abnormalities may only reflect the normal aging process of the disc.

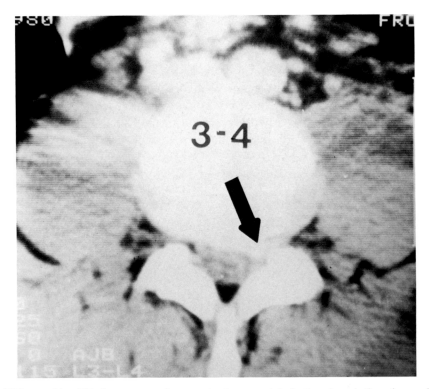

FIG. 5–16. CT-discogram demonstrating an L3-4 disc herniation (*arrow*). The contrast agent clearly shows accumulation anterior to the exiting nerve root.

Unlike CT discography, the MRI is non-invasive and painless and, as stated above, it is able to diagnose at least as accurately the degenerative changes associated with internal disc disruption. However, it cannot be over-emphasized that critical therapeutic decisions should not be based solely on the MRI appearance of early degenerative disc disease until definitive data are available correlating these early degenerative changes with an increased incidence of low back pain.

Despite these clinical reservations about the usefulness of this diagnostic study, many physicians feel strongly that CT discography has definite value in the workup of patients with long-standing low back pain. However, as discussed earlier, discography has always been controversial and continues to remain so. Only time will tell whether MRI will replace CT discography as the study of choice for those proponents of the internal disc disruption theory. If this does come to pass, the true value of the provocation test must then be re-assessed. The clinical information obtained from it in combination with the images of the CT discogram may therefore yield more information than the MRI alone. There is no consensus among physicians in any of these controversial areas and, unfortunately, there does not appear to be any consensus in sight.

Radionuclide scanning is useful in the lumbar spine primarily in patients suspected of having an invasive process involving the vertebrae. The routine bone scan is used primarily to detect primary or metastatic disease of the spine. In the presence of early primary or metastatic disease not yet evident on plain radiographs, a bone scan will often show increased uptake indicative of increased bone turnover (Fig. 5–17). Unfortunately, one of the diagnostic drawbacks of bone scanning is its inability to differentiate between cancerous lesions and other abnormalities resulting in a localized state of increased bone turnover.

The next most common condition diagnosed by radionuclide scanning other than primary or metastatic disease is vertebral osteomyelitis. For-

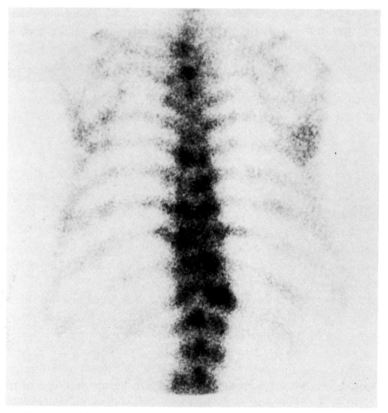

FIG. 5–17. A positive bone scan demonstrating multiple metastatic breast lesions throughout the thoracolumbar spine.

tunately additional diagnostic scans can often differentiate infectious processes from other abnormalities. Gallium and more recently indium scanning are quantitatively more sensitive to infectious processes than other invasive bony lesions.

Radionuclide scanning may also play a role in the diagnosis of several other non-invasive lesions affecting the lumbar spine. In patients with a spondylolytic defect and a recent onset of symptoms, it is often impossible to detect on plain radiographs a fresh fracture at the site of the lytic defect. A positive bone scan at the site of the lytic defect is supportive evidence that this lesion may be responsible for the painful symptoms (Fig. 5–18). A normal bone scan should warn the physician to look elsewhere for the etiology responsible for the patient's acute onset of pain.

In older patients with osteoporotic compression fractures of the vertebral body, it is often difficult to assess the age of the fracture on plain radiographs. Patients with acute symptoms and multiple levels of involvement may present a diagnostic dilemma when attempting to identify the cause of the acute symptoms. After 1 year the intensity of increased nuclide uptake begins to subside in most cases. It is often possible to differentiate the chronology of the fractures by the varied quantitative uptake on the bone scan.

Spinal pseudarthrosis may be identified by areas of increased uptake in an otherwise homogeneous fusion mass. Although the entire fusion mass may

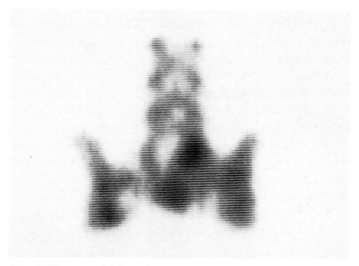

FIG. 5–18. A 17-year-old female gymnast with the acute onset of pain at the lumbosacral junction. Plain radiographs revealed only the presence of a unilateral spondylolysis. Bone scintigraphy confirmed the presence of an acute fracture.

show increased uptake for one year postoperative, established pseudarthroses, particularly those with detectable motion, will continue to show a marked increased uptake of radionuclide.

The use of thermography as a diagnostic tool has gained wide support from within and without the medical field. As a result of its easily interpreted colorful pattern of temperature changes, it has become a popular courtroom device in workers compensation and disability claims. The theoretic application of thermography rests on its ability to differentiate small changes in skin temperature along the areas of sciatic nerve distribution in the lower extremities. Unfortunately, there has been no scientific study that documents its reproducibility or efficacy. At this time it is recommended that no definitive diagnosis and certainly no treatment recommendation be based solely on the results of thermography until further scientific studies are available to document its clinical efficacy.

The routine use of electrodiagnostic studies in the diagnostic workup of the patient with low back pain remains controversial. An astute physician may often gain as much information from a thorough neurologic examination as from an expensive and painful electromyographic (EMG) study. Although these studies may play a role in determining the etiology of lower extremity neurologic loss, their use in the evaluation of the paravertebral muscles is certainly of little value. In fact, one study consisting of 70 patients with chronic low back pain found that the average EMG levels were statistically insignificant between the 40 patients having spinal surgery and those who had no surgery (1). Another study revealed similar findings when the clinical predictive value of paraspinal EMGs were evaluated in a group of patients with chronic low back pain and a group of asymptomatic patients performing routine tasks. There were no significant differences between either group in the paravertebral EMG activity (9). Overall there is no data that have shown that measuring electromyographic paravertebral muscle activity has any prognostic or diagnostic value in patients with low back pain.

Despite their lack of clinical usefulness in assessing the trunk musculature, the use of both electromyography and spinal evoked potentials may play a diagnostic role in patients with radicular symptoms. In the routine patient with a demonstrable neurologic deficit, they are not terribly useful and certainly no more helpful than a good clinical examination. However, the use of these studies may be beneficial in arriving at a diagnosis in patients with diabetic neuropathy, metabolic neuropathy, and demyelinating disorders.

In many patients with long-standing chronic low back pain and sciatica, the results of the electrodiagnostic studies may be somewhat equivocal and may only cloud the diagnostic picture. The use of these studies should be reserved for only the most difficult diagnostic cases. Unfortunately, the results may not contribute to a definitive diagnosis. These studies should never be used as the sole diagnostic study upon which a treatment regimen, particularly surgical intervention, is based.

Intraoperative spinal evoked potentials have been advocated as a guide to adequate neurologic decompression during surgery. Improvement in both latency and amplitude of the recorded potentials theoretically allows the surgeon insight into the adequacy of the decompression. However, in long-standing cases of neurologic compression, the spinal evoked potentials may never return to normal. Continuing surgical decompression in search of the "perfect wave" may result in an unnecessary radical decompression that is not indicated from a clinical or surgical perspective.

Routine blood and urine tests are not particularly helpful in the diagnostic workup in the patient with low back pain with or without sciatica unless there is some evidence of a systemic or metabolic etiology that may also involve the lumbar spine. The use of these studies should be reserved for those patients for whom there is clinical suspicion of an infectious, neoplastic, or metabolic abnormality affecting the spine. Otherwise, these tests will not routinely yield productive clinical data and will certainly not be cost effective.

REFERENCES

1. Ahern DK, Follick MJ, Council JR, et al: Reliability of lumbar paravertebral EMG assessment in chronic low back pain. *Arch Phys Med Rehabil* 1986;67:762–765.
2. Bell GR, Rothman RH, Booth RE, et al.: A study of computer-assisted tomography: II. Comparison of metrizamide myelography and computed tomography in the diagnosis of herniated lumbar disc and spinal stenosis. *Spine* 1984;9:552–556.
3. Bolender NF, Schonstrom NS, Spengler DM: Role of computed tomography and myelography in the diagnosis of central spinal stenosis. *J Bone Joint Surg* 1985;67A:240–246.
4. Bosacco SJ, Berman AT, Garbarino JL, et al: A comparison of CT scanning and myelography in the diagnosis of lumbar disc herniation. *Clin Orthop* 1984;190:124–128.
5. Frymoyer JW, Newberg A, Pope MH, et al: Spine radiographs in patients with low back pain: an epidemiological study in men. *J Bone Joint Surg* 1984;66A:1048–1055.
6. Herkowitz HN, Romeyn RL, Rothman RH: The indications for metrizamide myelography. *J Bone Joint Surg* 1983;65A:1144–49.
7. Jackson RP, Cain JE Jr, Jacobs RR, Cooper BR, McManus GE; The neuroradiographic diagnosis of lumbar herniated nucleus pulpous: II. A comparison of computed tomography (CT), myelography, CT-myelography, and magnetic resonance imaging. *Spine* 1989;14:1362–1367.
8. Masaryk TJ, Ross JS, Modic MT, et al: High resolution MR imaging of sequestered lumbar intervertebral discs. *A J R* 1988;150:1155–1162.
9. Miller DJ: Comparison of electromyographic activity in the lumbar paraspinal muscles of subjects with and without chronic low back pain. *Phys Ther* 1985;65:1347–1354.
10. Sachs BL, Vanharanta H, Spivey MA, et al.: Dallas discogram description: A new classification of CT/discography in low-back disorders. *Spine* 1987;12:287–294.

11. Schipper J, Kardaun JW, Braakman R, et al.: Lumbar disc herniation: Diagnosis with CT or myelography. *Radiology* 1987;165:227–231.
12. Schneiderman G, Flannigan B, Kingston S, Thomas J, Dillin WH, Watkins RG: Magnetic resonance imaging in the diagnosis of disc degeneration: Correlation with discography. *Spine* 1987;12:276–281.
13. Witt I, Vestergaard A, Rosenklint A: A comparative analysis of x-ray findings of the lumbar spine in patients with and without lumbar pain. *Spine* 1984;9:298–300.

6

Idiopathic Low Back Pain

The title for this chapter could just as easily have been "Mechanical Low Back Pain," "Lumbosacral Sprain," "Low Back Syndrome," "Lumbago," or a variety of other names commonly used to describe low back pain without associated sciatica, neurologic symptoms, or structural bony abnormalities. The ambiguity in arriving at a proper descriptive name for this disorder is due to our lack of insight into the pathophysiologic basis for low back pain. Perhaps *idiopathic low back pain* best describes the current state of our knowledge about the etiology of most cases of low back pain.

Despite a large number of diverse studies attempting to isolate the exact etiologic abnormality responsible for low back pain, there currently exists no acceptable proved etiology that accurately explains why 80% of the population experiences low back pain. Investigators have reported the results of both clinical and laboratory studies examining almost every anatomic structure comprising the lumbar spine, but none have conclusively been able to identify the causative abnormality. Theories attempting to incriminate the disc, facet joint complex, as well as the paraspinal muscles and supporting ligaments, as the structures responsible for the pain have not been successfully proved. Biochemical and ultrastructural studies of the intervertebral disc have also failed to identify the etiologic abnormality despite the recent popularization of the internal disc disruption theory. Similar histologic and histochemical studies have likewise failed to condemn the facet joint as the causative agent.

With the advent of increasingly sophisticated devices available to measure trunk strength and endurance, an extremely large number of studies continue to be reported that attempt to isolate the causation of low back pain. As with the disc and facet joint studies, a great deal of data has been generated but there remains no universally accepted etiology responsible for the low back pain among any of the strength parameters tested. There has been evidence that altered endurance of the trunk muscles may predispose the patient to having low back pain or sustaining a recurrence. Once again there is no common consensus that any of these measurements of isokinetic, isometric, or endurance strength are primarily responsible for the low back pain.

Attempts to correlate low back pain with degenerative changes on plain radiographs have also been unsuccessful. There is a wide discrepancy among studies over the significance of the degenerative radiographic abnormalities with most studies finding little correlation with any of the symptoms. Even in those studies with positive correlations, the findings do not appear to be consistent with the findings in other similar studies. Thus, there appears to be no better explanation for the low back pain based on the radiographic abnormalities than with the other proposed theories discussed above.

Despite our increasing ability to evaluate the histologic, biochemical, and mechanical aspects of the lumbar spine, the etiology for the most common of all musculoskeletal ailments continues to evade us. Perhaps the pain is due not only to one identifiable abnormality but a number of interrelated and interdependent abnormalities that may predispose an individual to having low back pain. With time, epidemiologic studies continue to identify risk factors associated with an increased incidence of low back pain. However, the true causation for low back pain remains elusive and any honest physician treating patients with low back pain must admit that idiopathic low back pain is an appropriately descriptive term for this exceedingly common ailment.

Even though there is no consensus on the exact etiology of low back pain, the history is just as important as in other ailments with a more clearly defined etiology. A careful history is extremely important in helping to identify those patients whose low back pain is caused by a more serious underlying abnormality and, on rare occasions, a life threatening one. Regardless of the fact that the vast majority of patients will present with a rather mundane and often boring history of pain in the lower back, the examining physician must never forget to ask the appropriate questions and always be aware of the slightest alteration in the usual clinical history of the patient with "garden variety" back pain.

The onset of lower back pain may be acute or insidious. Patients may or may not relate associated trauma with the acute onset of low back pain. It is quite common for patients to identify a particular incident of lifting, falling, twisting, or direct trauma at the onset of pain. Unless there is an associated bony fracture, it is very difficult to correlate the severity of the pain with the suspected severity of the trauma. Simple maneuvers such as bending forward to tie one's shoes often result in as much or more pain than that caused by a fall or lifting a very heavy object.

Despite the fact that the insignificance of the injury often does not seem to justify the severity of the pain, the most important piece of the history is the presence of any unusual aspects of the painful symptoms. Despite the presence of a precipitating incident, most idiopathic low back pain is relieved in the supine position particularly when the patient's hips and knees are flexed. The pain may often delay the patient's falling asleep but once asleep it is unusual for the patient to be awakened by the pain. Persistent, unrelenting pain that is not relieved by rest and awakens the patient from sleep is often associated with an invasive vertebral lesion such as a metastatic or primary tumor.

The patient with low back pain also does not typically have associated febrile episodes that may be indicative of a disc space infection or osteomyelitis. Any previous history of intravenous drug use should be questioned since a significant percentage of patients with vertebral osteomyelitis have a history of illicit drug abuse. The presence of any recent or past infectious diseases, particularly those of the genitourinary tract, should be sought in patients suspected of vertebral infection.

Elderly patients with metabolic bone disease, most commonly osteoporosis, may present with the acute onset of low back pain that is often associated with very minimal trauma. Minimal compression fractures are quite common in these patients. Plain radiographs often are not able to make a definitive diagnosis and bone scintigraphy is necessary. It must also be remembered that the presence of previous compression fractures in an elderly osteoporotic patient does not necessarily guarantee that all future fractures are due to the osteoporosis. Close scrutiny is necessary to avoid the concomitant presence of a metastatic or primary tumor superimposed on longstanding vertebral osteoporosis.

A history of low back pain is extremely common. The vast majority of patients with idiopathic low back pain will experience one or more recurrences in their lifetime and, as before, will probably not need extensive therapy or diagnostic testing. However, it is extremely important to determine whether there exists the possibility of any new pathologic process causing the new onset of pain.

The pain associated with idiopathic low back pain is often exacerbated by a variety of positions. Sitting seems to increase this type of pain more often than most other activities. It is quite common for the patient to experience an increase in pain when arising from the sitting or lying position to the standing position. Less frequently patients tend to complain about increased pain with standing in one position for long periods and even less frequently with walking. Lying in the supine or lateral position with the hips and knees flexed tends to alleviate or decrease the pain of idiopathic low back pain.

Sciatic pain with or without neurologic symptoms will be discussed in subsequent chapters. However, as discussed earlier in Chapter 3, true sciatic pain must be differentiated from referred pain. Once again, true sciatic pain must follow the radicular pattern of the sciatic nerve components. Referred pain into the buttocks, groin, and thigh must not be confused with true

sciatic pain. Patients with idiopathic low back pain do not have any associated neurologic deficits. Any patient with complaints of weakness, numbness, or bowel/bladder dysfunction should be assumed not to have idiopathic
low back pain and a more definitive etiology must be sought.

Positive physical findings associated with idiopathic low back pain are
frequently inconsistent and often completely absent. Palpation of the
spinous processes and/or adjacent paraspinal muscles may or may not elicit
pain. The pain may be localized to a small discrete muscular area frequently
referred to as a *trigger point* or it may be diffusely tender over a wide area of
the paraspinal muscles. It is not uncommon for small subcutaneous lipomatous masses adjacent to the inferior iliac spine to be tender to palpation. It is not clear why these fatty masses become painful. Conversely,
many patients may have no pain to palpation or percussion anywhere.

Although flexibility of the lumbar spine is often decreased in patients with
low back pain, the degree of restricted motion does not correlate in any way
with the severity of the pain. Pain on extension may emanate from increased
stresses on the facet joints and their capsule. Extremes of extension appear
to exacerbate facet joint abnormalities. However, the exact etiology of the
pain with extension is not known.

Idiopathic back pain may often limit forward flexion, but the limitation
may also be due to a variety of other ailments. Spondyloarthritis, although
not frequently seen, may commonly present with stiffness of the lumbar
spine. If there is clinical suspicion of spondyloarthritis, chest expansion
should be measured as well as manipulation of the sacroiliac joint in an
attempt to elicit pain. Altered joint motion of the hips and other peripheral
joints should also be checked.

Much more common than spondyloarthritis as a cause of restricted lumbar
spine motion and referred pain are tight hamstring muscles. Tight hamstring
muscles may limit forward flexion and produce pain in the posterior thigh
and buttocks when stretched. This may produce posterior thigh pain that is
often mistaken for sciatica. This is easily differentiated from true sciatica
because there is no radiation below the knee.

Idiopathic low back pain has no associated neurologic abnormalities. Any
patient with objective signs of neurologic irritability, motor or sensory loss
does not have idiopathic low back pain. Further diagnostic and clinical
studies are indicated since idiopathic low back pain should have none of the
above neurologic findings. The presence of any of these abnormalities
should alert the physician to search further for an intraspinal or structural
abnormality.

Just as the physical examination often reveals no insight into the cause of
the pain in patients with idiopathic low back pain, diagnostic studies are
equally as frustrating at arriving at a definitive diagnosis. As discussed ear-

lier, plain radiographs are not truly helpful at defining the cause of the pain unless there is another etiology. Primary and metastatic lesions, infection, and structural deformities such as spondylolisthesis may be demonstrated on plain radiographs when ordered by the astute physician who has noted an alteration of the normal history or physical examination from that usually presented by the patient with idiopathic low back pain. Although it has been shown that routine radiographs in patients with low back pain are not cost effective or diagnostically helpful, any suspicion on the part of the physician that a structural bony abnormality may be responsible for the pain should warrant ordering plain radiographs.

Unless there is a specific suspicion of an infectious process, inflammatory or metabolic disease affecting the spine, laboratory studies are not helpful. However, any suspicions arising out of the history and physical examination should be confirmed by the appropriate laboratory study in order to avoid inappropriate treatment or misdiagnosed idiopathic low back pain.

Idiopathic low back pain for the most part is a self-limited disease. The concept of low back pain as a disease may be somewhat flawed since at least 80% of the population sometime during their adult years will experience low back pain that will restrict their activities for a short period of time. If left untreated and to their own ways, the vast majority of patients will recover within a short period and be able to resume all normal unrestricted activities. In fact 70% of patients untreated for low back pain will be asymptomatic by 6 weeks. An additional 20% will be asymptomatic at 3 months. By 6 months, only 2% will still be experiencing symptoms and at 1 year after the onset of pain only 1% will still complain of symptoms.

Keeping these statistics in mind and realizing that the natural history of low back pain is quite benign if left untreated, it is truly amazing to realize the diverse types of treatment offered and the vast amounts of money spent on the treatment of idiopathic low back pain. The treatment of idiopathic low back pain has included gravity traction, massage therapy, trigger point injections, facet injections, electrical stimulation, ultrasound, manipulation, acupuncture, transcutaneous nerve stimulation (TENS), acupressure, bio-feedback, exercises, and surgery. Despite widespread claims of success for many of these proposed treatment modalities, there is a paucity of scientific data documenting their effect on the long-term outcome of patients with idiopathic low back pain.

It is best to divide these proposed treatments into passive and active modalities as well as invasive versus non-invasive techniques. Passive modalities are those in which the patient does not actively participate in the treatment. These would include ultrasound, massage, heat, cold, bracing, acupuncture, TENS, electrical stimulation, and a variety of manipulation and traction techniques. Many, and in fact most, provide immediate relief or a decrease in the painful symptoms. There is some limited evidence that several types of manipulation and traction may bring some consistent short-term relief of idiopathic low back pain (4). However, no scientific studies are available that document that any of these passive modalities influence the natural history of idiopathic low back pain. For the most part these passive treatment modalities have no role in the long-term management of idiopathic low back pain. Certainly, in a patient with the acute onset of idiopathic low back pain they may be useful in relieving the pain for a brief period to allow the patient to increase his or her activity level and begin to resume normal daily activities. However, until proved to be scientifically effective, these modalities are not recommended for long-term use.

In fact, many physicians feel that these treatments may be actually counterproductive. Patients often become dependent on these passive modalities to alleviate their pain, much as with any other psychological or physical addiction. In this manner, patients begin to rely on the physicians and therapists to "cure" their pain. Thus, patients shift the responsibility of getting over the symptoms of this self-limited ailment from themselves to their physicians or therapists, thereby allowing their participation in the recovery process to be unnecessarily passive and dependent. Obviously this type of behavior will often result in delayed improvement as well as mounting costs related to excessive use of treatment modalities still unproved to be effective in altering the natural history of patients with idiopathic low back pain.

The active treatment methods are those in which the patient actively participates in the treatment program. The most commonly used of these techniques are the various types of exercise programs for stretching and strengthening of the muscles in the anatomic region of the low back. For many years it was believed (and commonly practiced) that bedrest and restricted activities were the treatment of choice for idiopathic low back pain. It was not uncommon for patients to be put to bed for weeks on end with no attempt to return these patients to their normal daily activities.

More recently, epidemiologic studies have shown that this approach is not therapeutically effective and may be counterproductive. Studies have shown that 2 days of bedrest following the onset of pain was the optimal period of rest prior to increasing the patient's activity level (2). A rapid return to normal activities has been shown to shorten the episode of low back pain.

No longer is prolonged bedrest an acceptable way to treat low back pain. Likewise, prolonged bedrest with traction has also never been shown to alter the course of idiopathic low back pain. Simple physics reveals that the use of 30 to 40 pounds of pelvic traction is not even enough weight to overcome the force of the skin's friction on the bed. Otherwise, we would frequently see patients hanging by their weights off the end of the bed. If the applied weight is not enough to overcome the skin's friction, then what can we realistically expect these forces to be doing to the muscles, ligaments, joints, and discs of the lumbar spine. Perhaps the use of traction could be replaced by the use of hard restraints since both of these devices will effectively produce the same effect, i.e., keeping the patient tied to the bed. But as we now know, more than 2 days of this type of strict bed rest has no therapeutic benefit to patients with idiopathic low back pain.

As we continue to eliminate many of the long-standing but unproved methods of treatment for patients with idiopathic low back pain, physical fitness and active exercise participation remain two of the proved methods of affecting the natural history of idiopathic low back pain (1). Overall, physical fitness has been associated with a lower recurrence rate and shorter history of low back pain. Increased endurance and strength appear to have an effect on the outcome and natural history of the pain. This ties in nicely with the new-found knowledge that prolonged rest is contraindicated in the treatment of patients with idiopathic low back pain. It is generally accepted that these patients should start on a conditioning program as quickly as possible after the onset of symptoms. Initially, exercises should consist of mild stretching, progress to more intensive stretching, and finally to strengthening exercises. Patients with a prior history of idiopathic low back pain should attempt to begin stretching immediately at the onset of symptoms in hopes of preventing the so-called paraspinal spasm and tightening associated with idiopathic low back pain.

Once stretching exercises have begun and the pain has started to subside, strengthening exercises should be initiated. There are two schools of exercise therapy for the treatment of patients with idiopathic low back pain. Proponents of the Williams exercises believe that strengthening should involve the anterior group of trunk muscles with particular attention paid to the abdominal muscles. Proponents of the MacKenzie type of exercises believe that strengthening of the extensor or posterior muscle groups are the key to alleviating the pain.

Despite widespread claims of superiority by supporters of both groups of exercises, it does not appear that there is a significant difference in the clinical outcome of patients performing either flexion or extension exercises. According to data from one study comparing flexion and extension exercises, significant pain relief was seen in both groups, but there was no significant difference in the amount of pain relief found between the groups (3). Therefore, it seems that the patient's activity level and mobilization of the lumbar spine are more important than the exact type of exercise regime followed. It is probably best to teach patients a combined flexion and extension program to obtain the maximal stretching and strengthening effects of both, since neither appears to have a superior beneficial effect when compared to the other.

Participation in and popularization of back schools has grown rapidly since their first introduction in Sweden. The concept of the back school approach is to incorporate instruction and education of patients, demonstrating ways to reduce the symptoms, and, at the same time, actively engaging the patients' participation in proper body mechanics and progressive exercise programs. Since the first Swedish back school was opened, there have been a great number of back schools developed throughout the Western world. There now exists a wide variety of these programs custom designed for the local patient population. However, the growing diversity of the content of the programs makes clinical comparison and outcome analysis difficult. However, the back school approach does appear to be more effective when used in an industrial setting or with patients with the acute onset of symptoms. Back schools that stress prevention appear to reduce the number of injuries in the workplace and decrease the number of days lost by patients with acute injuries.

Although patients typically enjoy the back school and claim to find it helpful, particularly when there are no more than five sessions, its overall effectiveness on the natural history of idiopathic low back pain, particularly in those patients with long-standing symptoms, is not clearly established (5). Unfortunately, there is no consensus on the benefits of the back school approach for patients with idiopathic low back pain outside of the industrial setting.

Fortunately, there are far fewer invasive procedures advocated for the treatment of idiopathic low back pain. Trigger point injections at tender areas of muscular spasm have no scientific basis for altering the natural history of the low back pain. Regardless of whether the injection is performed with a local anesthetic with or without injectable steroids, no studies have shown any better results than with placebo injection or no treatment at all.

Medications used in the treatment of idiopathic low back pain should be kept to a minimum. There is virtually no role for the use of such strong and addictive medications such as Demerol, Dilaudid, Percodan, or Percocet. Even for patients in the acute phase when the intensity of the pain is at its height, the use of narcotic medication should be limited. There is rarely a need for any medication stronger than the more common codeine preparations. These should be restricted to the early phase of the symptoms and not used for prolonged periods of time. Most patients will have sufficient pain relief with the use of any number of the currently available nonsteroidal, anti-inflammatory medications to be able to eliminate the narcotic medications as quickly as possible.

Although the pharmaceutical manufacturers have spent a great deal of money on the development and marketing of numerous anti-inflammatory medications, there is little definitive evidence that these medications work any better in the treatment of idiopathic low back pain than the over-the-counter less expensive aspirin and other anti-inflammatory preparations.

As with stronger narcotic medications, there is likewise no role for muscle relaxants such as diazepam in the treatment of idiopathic low back pain. The best way to obtain muscle relaxation in the acute phase of the pain is to have the patient rest and restrict activities in combination with the appropriate pain medication. No evidence exists that centrally acting medications such as diazepam affects the recovery rate or natural history of idiopathic low back pain. A conscious effort should always be made by the physician to avoid any mood-altering or addictive medication when treating this benign musculoskeletal condition.

It is quite tempting to ascribe the long-standing chronic pain of the few patients with idiopathic low back pain who do not improve with time to an "unstable" motion segment. This is a very dangerous concept. In the absence of obvious structural deformity such as spondylolisthesis, spondylolysis, or other localized segmental deformities, there is no universal agreement on the definition or the way to properly diagnose segmental instability. Thus, fusion of a suspected "unstable" motion segment in an attempt to cure idiopathic low back pain will not result in an acceptable success rate. Even though at times surgery may appear to be the only remaining treatment alternative, there are no data available that validate a role for spinal fusion in the treatment of the patient with idiopathic low back pain. Until a great deal more is understood about the etiology of idiopathic low back pain, surgical intervention should be avoided at all costs.

REFERENCES

1. Cady LD, Jr, Thomas PC, Karawsky RJ: Program for increasing health and physical fitness of fire fighters. *J Occup Med* 1985;27:110–114.
2. Deyo RA, Diehl AK, Rosenthal M: How many days of bedrest for acute low back pain? *N Eng J Med* 1986;315:1064–1070.
3. Elnagger M, Nordin M, et al: The effects of spinal flexion and extension exercises on low back pain and spinal mobility in chronic mechanical low back pain patients. Presented at the North American Spine Society. July 26, 1988. Colorado Springs, Colo.
4. Haldeman S: Spinal manipulative therapy: A status report. *Clin Orthop* 1983;179:62–70.
5. Lankhorst GJ, Van de Stadt RJ, Volgelaar TW, et al: The effect of the Swedish Back School in chronic idiopathic low back pain: A prospective controlled study. *Scand J Rehabil Med* 1983;15:141–145.

7

Herniated Lumbar Disc

One of the most commonly confused concepts in all of lumbar spine disease is that a degenerative disc and a herniated disc are one and the same. All too frequently patients present with radiographs revealing only intervertebral disc space narrowing. They complain fearfully that their doctor claimed, "My x-rays showed a herniated disc." Despite the frequency of this scenario, we all know that the diagnosis of a herniated disc cannot be made or even suspected on the findings of plain radiographs since none of the soft tissue anatomy is visible on plain radiographs.

The presence of disc space narrowing on plain radiographs simply implies that there have been degenerative changes occurring in the disc that result in disc space narrowing. Whether the narrowing occurs chronologically as expected or is more accelerated in a younger individual, the presence of disc space narrowing should never be confused with a true herniated disc. The histologic and biochemical changes occurring in the degenerative disc are distinctly different from those found in a disc herniation.

With the normal aging process and subsequent disc space narrowing, bulging of the posterior annulus typically occurs. As our ability to visualize intraspinal anatomy has improved with myelography, CT scanning, and now MRI, it has become commonplace to describe the bulging annulus of the degenerative disc, particularly in spinal stenosis, as herniated. However, an understanding of the pathophysiology of the normal aging process of the lumbar motion segment will quickly clarify any confusion of a bulging degenerative disc with a true disc herniation.

In a true lumbar disc herniation (as opposed to simply a degenerative lumbar disc), there are actually fractures or discrete disruptions in the normal concentric structure of the posterior annulus. The extent of the annular disruption to a large degree determines the type and severity of the disc herniation.

For many years lumbar disc herniations were depicted in both lay and medical publications as if the herniation were caused by a "jelly doughnut" type leakage or a defect in the outer annulus allowing for leakage of the nuclear material, much like squeezing a jelly doughnut and watching the jelly escape (Fig. 7–1). As more sophisticated histologic and pathologic

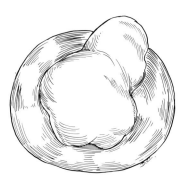

FIG. 7–1. Although the "jelly doughnut" depiction of a herniated disc is still widely used, a wide variety of histologic and pathologic studies have shown definitively that this is not a true representation of the pathologic anatomy responsible for a herniated disc. The perpetuation of the "jelly doughnut" theory is responsible for a variety of unfounded diagnostic and treatment modalities.

studies have shown, the lumbar disc herniation has been clearly shown not to be like jelly leaking from the nucleus but, in actuality, it consists of displaced fragments of annular and nuclear material, which are quite firm and fibrous and not jelly-like as previously depicted (12). Unfortunately, this widely accepted and commonly misunderstood concept has led to a variety of erroneous methods of treatment and diagnosis. This diagrammatic depiction of the lumbar disc herniation should forever be laid to rest to prevent further generations from misunderstanding the true pathophysiology of the lumbar disc herniation.

A variety of names and classifications has been used to describe the various types of disc herniations. These include such terms as *ruptured, slipped, protruded, bulging, extruded*, and *sequestered*. Unfortunately, there is no universal acceptance of any of these terms describing a disc herniation. Despite this lack of agreement on descriptive terms, it is easiest to understand and classify the type of herniation based on the pathoanatomic changes.

A partial disruption or tear of the outer posterior annular fibers allows for a localized bulging or protrusion of the disc. When this occurs, anterior to an exiting nerve root, symptoms of unilateral sciatica may be present. This type of herniation in which there is only a partial disruption of the posterior annulus is known as a bulging or protruded disc herniation (Fig. 7–2A). A complete disruption of the posterior annulus with more significant protrusion of the annular material but still confined to the disc space by the intact posterior longitudinal ligament is called an extruded disc herniation (Fig. 7–2B). A sequestered disc herniation is similar to an extruded disc hernia-

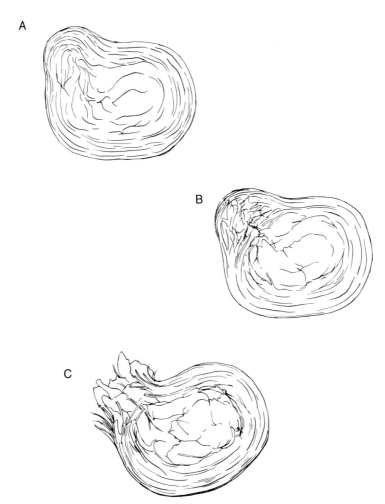

FIG. 7–2. A: A bulging or protruded disc may cause nerve root compression, but the outer annular layers are only partially disrupted and the posterior longitudinal ligament remains intact. **B:** Complete disruption of the posterior annulus will result in an extruded disc herniation if the posterior longitudinal ligament remains intact. **C:** Complete disruption of the annulus and posterior longitudinal ligament may result in a sequestered disc herniation. Migration of the fragment may occur as there are no remaining intact anatomic structures to keep the herniated annular fragments in continuity with the rest of the disc.

tion except that the posterior longitudinal ligament is disrupted allowing for the possibility of migration or separation of the disrupted annular fragments away from the disc space (Fig. 7–2C). Preoperative studies may not consistently be able to differentiate the three types of herniation. This is particularly true in attempting to differentiate a large bulging disc from an extruded disc herniation or a large extruded disc herniation from a sequestered fragment that has not migrated. As discussed previously, the differentiation of these various types of disc herniation is being made easier as the MRI images become more technologically sophisticated.

Even though it is becoming easier to visualize lumbar disc herniations with ever-increasing technical advances, it is important for the physician to realize that the vast majority of patients seen with low back pain will not have a herniated disc and even fewer will ever need surgical intervention. As discussed earlier, of all those patients presenting with low back pain only 10–12% will complain of sciatica as well. To further deter any eager spinal surgeons, at best only 2% and, more realistically less than 1%, of all patients with low back pain will ever require a surgical procedure.

In the United States roughly 10 million people experience low back pain yearly (2). According to one source, much less than 1%, or approximately 256,000 people, will require any type of spinal surgery (8). Out of these 256,000 operations approximately 188,000 will be lumbar decompressions for a herniated lumbar disc. Obviously the vast majority of patients presenting with low back pain and sciatica will never need any type of surgical treatment.

Lumbar disc herniation appears to be more common in males than in females. The most common age group of patients presenting with sciatica secondary to a herniated lumbar disc is the fifth decade. Even though the large majority of patients with symptoms due to a herniated lumbar disc are between the ages of 20 and 55, there are occasionally patients in their teens as well as in their later years that will present with symptoms caused by a herniated lumbar disc.

Younger patients in their teens suffering from a herniated disc present with surgical pathology distinctly different from their older counterparts. Instead of disc material containing principally annular fragments and lesser amounts of nuclear material, adolescent disc herniations frequently result in fragments of annulus and fractured portions of the vertebral endplate. The pathophysiology of this phenomenon distinguishing it from the older patient with a lumbar disc herniation is poorly understood. The potential presence of this pathologic anomaly should be recognized both on the preoperative studies as well as at the time of surgery.

As with adolescents, it is as equally infrequent to have a true lumbar disc herniation past the seventh decade. By this time the normal aging process has significantly changed the histologic appearance of the lumbar disc so that the incidence of actual disc herniations as compared to degenerative bulging of the posterior annulus is relatively uncommon.

Patients with a herniated lumbar disc typically present with unilateral sciatic pain. It is crucial to differentiate true sciatic pain from the referred pain that is so common with idiopathic low back pain. Many patients with sciatica from a herniated lumbar disc may or may not have concomitant low back pain. However, even in the absence of low back pain patients will complain of buttock pain radiating into the lower extremity below the knee.

The onset of symptoms may or may not be associated with a traumatic event. The sciatic symptoms may be present initially or follow a brief or prolonged period of back pain alone. Unfortunately there is no characteristic presentation in the typical patient with a herniated lumbar disc, but the common denominator for the proper diagnosis is the sciatic symptoms.

As stated above, the sciatic pain is almost always unilateral. It is highly unusual to have bilateral sciatic pain due to a herniated lumbar disc. On rare occasion an extremely large herniation, particularly in the midline, may cause bilateral sciatic signs and symptoms. However, the examining physician must realize that bilateral sciatic symptoms are quite atypical for the patient with a herniated lumbar disc and a thorough investigation into the possibility of another intraspinal lesion presenting with bilateral sciatica is usually warranted.

Cauda equina syndrome is often accompanied by bilateral sciatic pain. Patients with compression of the distal neural elements of the cauda equina may present with bladder and/or bowel deficits. These may present initially as urinary retention or later by overflow incontinence accompanied by frequent small volume urination. In addition to the bladder dysfunction, there may be sensory changes in the perineum or perianal skin as well as loss of anal sphincter tone and normal reflexes.

Cauda equina syndrome as well as progressive neurologic deficit of the affected lower extremity should be considered an emergency. Unlike the vast majority of patients presenting with sciatic symptoms, these patients should have either an immediate MRI or myelogram to rule out the possibility of cauda equina compression due to a large disc herniation or other intraspinal mass. If MRI or myelography reveals the presence of an intraspinal compression correlating to the clinical presentation, immediate surgical intervention is necessary. Fortunately, cauda equina syndrome is infrequently seen, but it is always imperative to question each patient about the presence of bowel or bladder symptoms even in the absence of lower extremity sciatic pain. Failure to properly diagnose and treat a patient with cauda equina syndrome may result in permanent neurologic dysfunction that may have easily been avoided with timely and appropriate care.

The radicular pattern of the sciatic pain may afford some insight into the exact level of involvement. A disc herniation at the L3–4 level typically presents with pain radiating into the distribution of the L4 nerve root. The pain and numbness is usually located on the medial aspect of the knee. The L3–4 disc herniations comprises less than 10% of all disc herniations found in the lumbar spine. The remaining 90% or more are evenly distributed between the L4–5 and L5–S1 disc. Herniation of the L4–5 disc with compression of the L5 nerve root results in pain and sensory complaints over the lateral calf and first dorsal web space. Herniation of the L5–S1 disc compressing the S1 nerve root causes pain radiating to the lateral foot and sole with sensory complaints in the same distribution.

On occasion, a very lateral disc herniation may also cause compression of the most proximal nerve root as well as the nerve root at the level of the herniation. Likewise a large medial herniation may cause impingement of the next distal nerve root resulting in symptoms referrable to two anatomic levels. This is quite common with a large L4–5 herniation causing symptoms not only referrable to the L5 nerve root but also the S1 nerve root (Fig. 7–3).

Patients with a herniated lumbar disc often report an increase in pain with any type of prolonged or increased activity. Sitting typically results in more pain than standing or walking. Patients often complain that driving a car is the worst activity for pain provocation. Unlike the radicular pain of spinal stenosis, patients with sciatic pain due to a herniated lumbar disc frequently find walking to be much less pain provoking than sitting. Most patients find that lying with the hips and knees flexed will alleviate or decrease their symptoms.

As with any diagnostic dilemma, the physical examination should provide information to confirm or deny the presumptive diagnosis arrived at from the history. Physical inspection of the spine and trunk of the patient with a herniated lumbar disc often demonstrates listing to one side or the other. This is commonly referred to as a *sciatic scoliosis* (Fig. 7–4). Radiographs often show a functional scoliosis without the typical rotational changes found in structural scoliosis. Alleviation of the pain will also alleviate the scoliosis. Attempts have been made to localize the type and location of the herniation by the direction of the list. Unfortunately, none of these theories have been shown to be consistently predictable.

Forward flexion in the upright position will usually cause radiation of the sciatic pain into the affected leg. It is important to differentiate the referred pain so common in idiopathic low back pain from true sciatic pain. The pain with flexion with a herniated disc is in contrast to spinal stenosis pain in which extension provokes the radicular pain that is actually alleviated by forward flexion. Patients with tight hamstring muscles complain of ham-

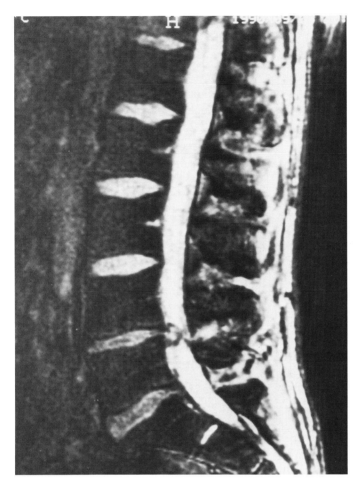

FIG. 7–3. A large L4-5 herniation extending toward the midline may also cause impingement of the S1 root as well as the L5 nerve root. Thus, a patient such as this may present with signs and symptoms emanating from two nerve roots instead of one.

string pain on forward flexion and this also must be carefully differentiated from true sciatic pain.

The motor examination and sensory examination should reveal objective signs of specific nerve root involvement. It is possible to have more than one root involved in a lumbar disc herniation, but even in these cases there should be easily diagnosed objective findings referrable to the specific affected nerve root. If the motor and sensory abnormalities do not conform to the typical nerve root distribution expected, other diagnostic possibilities should be entertained. It must be remembered that individual nerve root

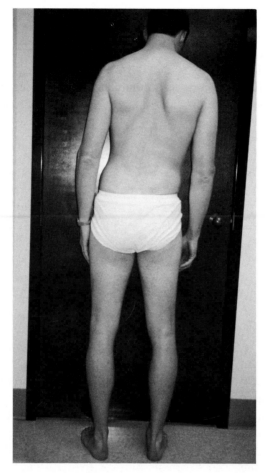

FIG. 7–4. Patients with a herniated disc will often present with a list and a "sciatic" scoliosis. The list and scoliosis will typically be corrected with alleviation of the painful symptoms.

involvement results in specific motor and sensory changes that have been previously discussed. Deviation from this typical anatomic presentation does not bode well for a presumptive diagnosis of a herniated lumbar disc.

Asymmetry, or absence of the knee or ankle jerk, is also strong evidence of specific nerve root compression. However, with any motor and sensory change, the reflex abnormalities must conform to the suspected nerve root involved. Herniation of the L3–4 disc may cause asymmetry of the knee jerk. Herniation of the L5–S1 disc as well as a large L4–5 disc herniation may result in asymmetry of the ankle jerk. The presence of any pathologic reflex changes such as a positive Babinski reflex or clonus is strong evidence that there is upper motor neuron pathology and that the diagnosis of a herniated lumbar disc should be discarded.

Patients with a herniated lumbar disc characteristically present with unilateral neural irritability. This is manifested on the physical examination by a positive straight leg raising test, contralateral straight leg raising, or bowstring test. It is highly unusual for any of these tests to be positive bilaterally. It cannot be over-emphasized that referred pain or hamstring tightness should never be confused with true sciatic pain.

The patient with an ideal herniated lumbar disc will present with all of the above findings of discrete and specific motor, sensory, and reflex changes attributable to irritation of one particular nerve root. Unfortunately, as with any ailment, patients with ideal symptoms are in the minority. Most patients will not have every objective abnormality possible. In fact, most patients will present with only several of the above abnormalities indicative of nerve root compression. The important thing to remember is that the more positive objective findings present during the physical examination, the stronger the evidence to support the diagnosis based on a herniated lumbar disc. The more findings, the stronger the case, and the better the likelihood that the patient will respond well to appropriate treatment. The fewer the findings, the weaker the case and the less likelihood that the patient will respond to appropriate treatment, particularly surgical intervention.

Once a tentative diagnosis is reached based upon the history and physical examination, radiographic confirmation is needed before a definitive diagnosis can be made. Unless there is evidence of cauda equina syndrome with concomitant bladder or bowel dysfunction or progressive neurologic deficit, diagnostic studies should be delayed until 4 to 6 weeks have passed after the onset of symptoms. Most patients by that time will have improved to the point at which diagnostic studies are not necessary. By waiting this period of time with patients without significant neurologic deficit, a great number of unnecessary and expensive studies may be avoided. However, a patient with significant neurologic involvement should be considered an emergency and immediate MRI or myelography should be performed followed by the appropriate treatment.

Plain radiographs are not particularly helpful in the diagnosis of the herniated lumbar disc even though disc space narrowing indicative of degenerative disc disease is often misdiagnosed as a herniated lumbar disc. It must be remembered that a herniated lumbar disc is a soft tissue abnormality involving the intervertebral disc and the affected nerve root. Neither of these structures are visible on plain radiagraphs.

Although there is no universal agreement on the best diagnostic test to confirm a herniated lumbar disc, the MRI as it continues to improve with technologic advances, is becoming the procedure of choice in the diagnosis of the herniated lumbar disc. Many of the invasive disadvantages of both myelography and CT scanning have been overcome with the MRI. However, the physician must be aware of the sensitivity of the MRI to detect very early degenerative changes taking place in the intervertebral disc and must avoid improper overdiagnosis. This can be accomplished only by the appropriate correlation of the patient's history, physical findings, and appearance of the MRI. It can never be overstated, "Treat patients, not x-rays or MRI pictures."

Failure to demonstrate a disc herniation on the MRI may then warrant additional diagnostic testing. Discography, particularly CT discography, has gained popularity in difficult diagnostic situations. Unfortunately, there still exists a great deal of controversy over the validity of its use and it is generally not used as the sole indication for surgical intervention. The same holds true for electromyographic studies. These studies in routine cases are probably just as good as a careful neurologic examination and certainly less painful and expensive. In patients with an unclear diagnosis, electrodiagnostic studies may be more helpful in the diagnosis of a primary neurologic disorder than of a compressive lesion such as a herniated lumbar disc. In any case, surgical intervention should not be based solely on the electromyographic studies alone without additional diagnostic corroboration.

Routine laboratory studies are not helpful nor indicated in the workup of the patient suspected of having a herniated lumbar disc. The same holds true for other studies such as bone scintigraphy or thermography.

Once a tentative diagnosis is established, the initial treatment is not unlike that for patients with idiopathic low back pain. In the absence of cauda equina syndrome or progressive neurologic deficit, patients should initially be treated with a brief period of bedrest. Patients commonly find maximum relief lying with the hips and knees flexed, thereby avoiding stretching the sciatic nerve and its component nerve roots.

Complete or strict bedrest is advisable for several days only. At that time, patients should attempt to increase their activity levels as much as tolerated. Activity level should be based on the patient's pain level. As the pain subsides the activity level should increase. There are no data showing any long-term benefit of prolonged bedrest in alleviating the pain or disability caused by a herniated lumbar disc. At this time there is no scientific basis for recommending prolonged bedrest.

Despite years of tradition, the same lack of supportive scientific data are true for the use of traction. There is no evidence that short- or long-term traction of any type conclusively shortens the natural history or long-term outcome of the patient with a herniated lumbar disc. Thus, as with prolonged bedrest, there currently is no role for traction in the treatment of the patient with a herniated lumbar disc.

A large number of manipulative techniques have been advocated in the treatment of the patient with a herniated lumbar disc. These have included passive manipulations commonly performed by chiropractors and self-manipulation and traction techniques. Limited evidence is available that lends some support to the use of manipulation in affecting the short-term relief of symptoms (3). However, outside of short-term pain reduction, there is no data that has shown that any of the manipulation modalities are able to influence the long-term course of the patient with a herniated lumbar disc.

Unlike patients with idiopathic low back pain, exercises have not been able to influence the outcome of the patient with a herniated lumbar disc. Despite claims of successful treatment by proponents of flexion and particularly extension exercises, there are no data that have definitively shown any improved long-term results with either exercise regime. Even though there is no scientific evidence that exercises will influence the long-term outcome of patients with a documented herniated lumbar disc, for those patients showing clinical improvement (as most do), exercises should be added to their daily activities to improve flexibility and overall physical conditioning. Exercises that are known to positively influence low back pain should be recommended, even though their ineffectiveness in influencing the symptoms due to a herniated lumbar disc is understood.

The use of passive modalities such as ice, heat, ultrasound, massage, and electrical stimulation have no therapeutic value in shortening the long-term course of symptoms due to a herniated lumbar disc. By themselves, these modalities have no role in treating the patient with a herniated lumbar disc. On occasion they may be helpful in the short-term relief of the symptoms, and, thereby, allow the improving patient to increase his or her activity level. However, these modalities should never be relied upon as the definitive treatment, nor should they be used for prolonged periods of time because of their expense and the patient's tendency to rely on these passive modalities as the only source of pain relief.

The physician should follow the same guidelines for the use of medications as those used for the treatment of acute symptoms of idiopathic low back pain. The prolonged use of addictive narcotic medications should be avoided at all costs. As soon as possible, narcotic medications should be discontinued and the patient started on non-narcotic pain relievers. A wide array of nonsteroidal anti-inflammatory medications are now available for use with this type of patient. It is not clearly established that any of these medications are any more effective than aspirin, even though they are certainly more expensive. Aspirin, acetaminophen, or over-the-counter ibuprofen should be prescribed before resorting to the more expensive prescription nonsteroidal anti-inflammatory medications.

Although muscle relaxant medications are commonly used in treating the patient with a herniated lumbar disc, their usefulness in the treatment of sciatic pain due to a herniated lumbar disc has never truly been established. There is probably little role for these medications in the patient with sciatica, particularly those medications of the addictive narcotic variety.

The use of both intravenous and oral colchicine in the treatment of sciatic pain caused by a herniated lumbar disc has remained controversial over the years. It appears that intravenous administration yields better results than does oral colchicine, but its method of action has never been well understood. Although proponents of intravenous colchicine still widely advocate its use, critics continue to argue that it has no influence on the natural course of the pain associated with a herniated lumbar disc. Until further data or prospective trials are available, the use of intravenous or oral colchicine cannot wholeheartedly be recommended.

The use of epidural steroids in the treatment of the patient suffering from sciatic pain due to both spinal stenosis and a herniated lumbar disc has remained controversial. Prospective and retrospective studies have shown that the use of epidural steroids does not have any long-term effectiveness in the treatment of the sciatic symptoms due to spinal stenosis or a herniated lumbar disc (1,7). Only approximately 50% of patients get any significant long-term relief after the use of epidural steroids. Unfortunately, this is probably no better than treatment with a placebo.

Despite this apparent lack of long-term effectiveness, a significant number of patients do experience short-term relief of their sciatic pain with epidural steroids. Unfortunately, in the majority of patients the pain relief is not prolonged. Although evidence suggests that epidural steroids have no true long-term effectiveness, they are still widely used. Their widespread use will most likely continue until further studies confirm or repudiate the results of studies such as the ones cited above.

It may appear that, based on the above information, there is little that one may due to actively influence the natural history of the patient with a herniated lumbar disc. Unfortunately, this may be true. Certainly none of the modalities discussed above has had any significant long-term effect on these patients. Fortunately for the vast majority of patients, the natural history is one of continued improvement over the first 4 to 6 weeks. For those 90–95% of patients who do improve and become asymptomatic, it is poorly understood from a pathophysiologic basis why this occurs. Until we better understand what happens anatomically and physiologically to allow improvement and resolution of the sciatic symptoms, we may not be able to offer much more than guided benign neglect.

For those patients who have not improved by 6 to 8 weeks and who have a documented disc herniation on diagnostic testing that correlates with their clinical presentation, surgical intervention should be considered. Patients with neurologic loss and severe sciatic pain appear to have a better outcome if surgery is performed within 3 months of the onset of symptoms. Delaying the surgery past 12 weeks appears to compromise the clinical results (9).

The time-honored method of surgical treatment is surgical disc excision. For many years this was a rather involved surgical undertaking with a formal laminectomy performed and painstaking attempts to remove the entire disc carried out. Over time, this rather zealous approach has been refined and simplified to what is now referred to as a limited surgical discectomy. Although by tradition surgical discectomy is often referred to as a laminectomy, a formal laminectomy is almost never required to perform a limited discectomy and laminectomy is never an appropriate descriptive term for the surgical procedure.

When planning a limited surgical discectomy, two important objectives should be considered. The first is adequate anatomic exposure allowing the surgeon clear visualization of the disc herniation and the affected neurologic structures. Clear visualization of the neurologic structures is critical to avoid unnecessary complications that will certainly arise if one cannot clearly see the nerve roots and dural sac in the operative field. The second objective is to minimize the surgical trauma and avoid altering the normal anatomy as much as possible. In this manner potential postoperative instability can be avoided as well as excessive epidural scarring. A fine balance between adequate exposure and minimal surgical trauma can easily be attained by following the general guidelines of a limited surgical discectomy and avoiding a formal laminectomy and excessively vigorous disc excision.

The procedure is best performed with the patient in the prone knee-chest position with the abdomen hanging free to minimize congestion of the epidural veins. A midline incision is made between the adjacent spinous processes of the affected disc. The paraspinal muscles are stripped subperiostally with care being taken to avoid exposure of the facet joint capsule. Only the symptomatic side is exposed, leaving the contralateral side as well as the interspinous and supraspinous ligaments undisturbed. Self-retraining retractors are used to retract the elevated paraspinal muscles.

The ligamentum flavum is cleaned of all adherent tissue and excised from its inferior attachment to the lamina. If there is any doubt about the appropriate disc level, an intraoperative radiograph should be performed prior to removal of the ligamentum flavum. Excision of the wrong disc is unforgiveable and easily avoided.

After excision of the ligamentum flavum from its inferior attachment to the lamina, the lateral half of the ligamentum flavum on the affected side is removed with a Kerrison rongeur. It is important to remove enough ligamentum flavum laterally to gain visualization of the exiting nerve root (Fig. 7–5).

Remembering that the undersurface of the facet joint capsule is formed by the ligamentum flavum will facilitate visualization of the nerve root. At the

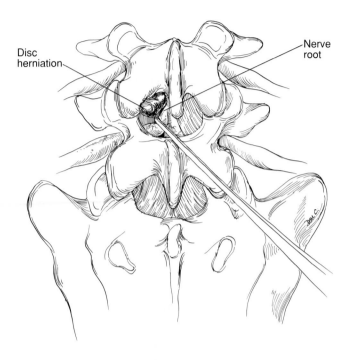

Disc
herniation

Nerve
root

FIG. 7–5. Clear visualization of the nerve root is critical before proceeding with the disc excision. Failure to visualize the nerve root, particularly at the L3–4 or L4–5 levels, is most often due to inadequate removal of the lateral extent of the ligamentum flavum. Once the nerve root has been identified, it can be safely retracted for exposure and entrance into the disc space.

L3–4 and L4–5 levels, it is often necessary to remove a small portion of the inferior margin of the superior lamina as well as undercutting the superior facet and lateral recess to gain adequate exposure of the nerve root. It is never necessary to perform a facetectomy and rarely necessary to remove more than a small portion of the lamina.

At this point inspection of the disc should not be done until the exiting nerve root and dural sac are clearly visualized. When there is difficulty encountered in visualizing the nerve root because of poor exposure or displacement by a disc fragment, its constant relationship to the pedicle should be kept in mind. If the nerve root cannot be identified, palpation or visualization of the pedicle will often facilitate localization of the nerve root as it courses inferior to the pedicle and out the foramen.

Once the nerve root has been identified, it should be gently retracted with a nerve root retractor and the underlying disc inspected. Correlation of the gross appearance of the disc and its appearance on preoperative diagnostic studies should be done. Prior to entering the disc space, a thorough search proximally and distally should be done to ensure that no sequestered fragments are overlooked. In the absence of a tear in the annulus and posterior longitudinal ligament, a single horizontal incision should be made through the attenuated annulus and posterior ligament. Multiple annular incisions or criss-cross incisions should be avoided to minimize annular disruption and scarring anterior to the nerve root.

With the nerve retracted, pituitary rongeurs should be used to remove any completely or partially sequestered fragments. The disc space should then be entered with the pituitary rongeurs and any loose fragments removed. No attempt should be made to remove excessive amounts of disc material or endplate. One must keep in mind that the purpose of the surgery is to decompress the nerve root irritated by the displaced disc material. Removing normal intra-discal material and curetting the cartilagenous endplates does nothing to achieve this goal.

Following evacuation of the herniated disc material, the nerve root should be checked for any remaining impingement along its course through the lateral recess. Lateral recess stenosis is much more common at the L4–5 space than at the L5–S1 space. It is not uncommon, particularly in older individuals, to have lateral recess stenosis due to hypertrophic spurring of the superior facet. This is easily removed by undercutting the ligemantum flavum and facet joint with a small Kerrison rongeur that will not affect the integrity or stability of the facet joint. A facetectomy is never indicated.

The use of fat grafts to prevent epidural scar formation is not universally accepted, although it still remains the best material to prevent postoperative scarring. Gel foam with or without local steroids is contraindicated because of experimental evidence suggesting that postoperative scarring is actually increased.

Postoperatively the patient should be ambulating the same day as the surgery. The usual postoperative hospitalization varies between 2 and 4 days. Patients should be encouraged to resume their normal activities as quickly as comfort allows. The only restriction should be excessive repetitive bending, rotation, and lifting for the first 3 weeks. At 3 weeks postoperative, patients should be started on a flexion and extension exercise program to enhance flexibility and begin strengthening.

This method of surgical disc excision is the standard against which all other methods of invasive treatment must be weighed. In noncompensation patients operated upon within the first 12 weeks of symptoms, approximately 90% of patients should have a good result and, by 8 weeks, they should have resumed the vast majority of all normal activities.

Proponents of microdiscectomy claim that the use of the microscope to perform the discectomy allows for better anatomic visualization, less surgical trauma, and a quicker return to normal activities. Opponents of microscopic discectomy claim that the use of the microscope does not allow enough visualization to adequately locate sequestered fragments, it restricts access to adequate lateral recess decompression, and it carries a higher infection rate. The use of the microscope has not been definitively shown to improve the overall clinical results of patients undergoing surgical discectomy. In fact one study has shown that the clinical outcome and the ability and speed to return to work is statistically indistinguishable in two groups of patients undergoing either a limited surgical discectomy or a microdiscectomy (5).

Microdiscectomy is almost identical in technique to the limited surgical discectomy except that many of the instruments used are microsurgical instruments. It is difficult to understand how a well-performed limited surgical discectomy differs from a microdiscectomy other than the addition of microscopic magnification. According to the conclusions of the above study, the addition of magnification does not appear to produce a significant clinical advantage over limited surgical discectomy. At this time microdiscectomy certainly appears to be an excellent surgical alternative to a limited surgical discectomy. However, it should be viewed as only that, an alternative, and not a clinically superior procedure.

One of the more controversial methods of treating the patient with a herniated lumbar disc over the last decade has been chemonucleolysis. Chymopapain is a proteolytic enzyme obtained from the papaya plant. It is injected under fluoroscopic control into the center of the herniated disc. The enzymatic action of the chymopapain allows desiccation of the disc with subsequent collapse and narrowing by altering the mucopolysaccharide's ability to bind water.

After FDA approval in the early 1980s, the use of chymopapain soared. The first year, almost 75,000 cases of chemonucleolysis were performed in the United States alone. Success rates consistently averaged 75% in a variety of studies performed shortly after its release. One long-term study following patients over 10 years found no significant differences in patients undergoing chemonucleolysis or surgery on final follow-up (10).

Unfortunately, within a few years of its release a large number of complications began to be reported (6). Initially anaphylaxis was the most significant complication. However, with the introduction of both serum and skin testing to detect allergic individuals, anaphylactic reaction has not been a significant problem. It was also recognized that the incidence of anaphylaxis was significantly higher when general anesthesia was used. Chemonucleolysis should be performed only with the patient awake in order to avoid any potential increase in anaphylactic reactions.

Shortly after the anaphylactic reactions were for the most part eliminated, reports of severe neurologic reactions began to surface. Initially chemonucleolysis was recommended to be performed after discographic contrast was injected into the disc to insure proper needle placement and to confirm that a disc herniation was present. A retrospective review of these complications, mostly involving patients with symptoms consistent with a transverse myelitis, found consistent evidence of intradural injection of both contrast agent and chymopapain (6). Subsequent animal studies confirmed these suspicions. The injudicious injection of chymopapain and contrast agent has been associated with a high incidence of paraplegia and transverse myelitis. Shortly after this discovery, discography was no longer recommended and in fact was contraindicated at the time of chymopapain injection.

With the appearance of these neurologic complications, the use of chymopapain dropped off almost as quickly as it rose. Although chymopapain appears to be relatively safe if done as recommended under local anesthesia, without discography and with both anteroposterior (AP) and lateral confirmation of proper needle placement prior to injection, it still has a success rate of only approximately 75%. This is clinically inferior to both microdiscectomy and limited surgical discectomy. With its rocky clinical course, it is unlikely that chemonucleolysis will ever attain the popularity it once had.

Clinical trials with another injectable enzyme, collagenase, followed shortly after chymopapain. In the wake of the complications surrounding chymopapain and reports of complications specific to collagenase, collagenase never attained the popularity of chymopapain and currently remains under investigation only.

The latest innovation and alternative to surgical disc excision is percutaneous discectomy. Percutaneous discectomy was first performed through a posterolateral approach with modified pituitary rongeurs introduced through a trochar into the disc space under fluoroscopic control. Removal of disc material from the central portion of the disc was then accomplished with the modified pituitary rongeurs.

Since the introduction of percutaneous discectomy, this has evolved into a more technically sophisticated and automated procedure. The automated device utilized to evacuate the disc material is introduced through a trochar approximately $2^{1}/_{2}$ mm in diameter. The procedure is performed with the patient awake under local anesthesia and fluoroscopic control. The newly devised automated tool has a biting device set several millimeters back from the tip, which repetitively bites small amounts of disc material. The material is then removed from the disc space by a suction-irrigation system.

The pathophysiologic theory upon which success of this system is based is the evacuation of a central defect in the disc into which the bulging disc may then collapse, thereby decompressing the affected nerve root. In theory this sounds quite appealing, but closer inspection into the pathophysiology of the lumbar disc herniation reveals that it has little validity. If disc herniations were truly like the traditional jelly doughnut representation, then this device would work well. Unfortunately, evacuating a central hole will not allow the fractured displaced fragments to collapse back into the hold as if they were oozing jelly.

Early series of percutaneous discectomy were reporting exceedingly good results comparable and, in some cases superior, to the results of microdiscectomy or limited surgical discectomy. Compared to chemonucleolysis, there were no reports of significant complications. The hospital stay was minimal and often eliminated by performing the procedure on an outpatient basis. However, as time passed, the earlier reports of success with percutaneous discectomy are now being contradicted. One later multicenter study reported only a 55% return-to-work rate following percutaneous discectomy in noncompensation patients (4). With success rates in this range, more time and additional data are needed before percutaneous discectomy can be considered a viable alternative to either microdiscectomy or limited surgical discectomy.

For many years, spinal fusion was a routine part of every discectomy performed. However, if we look closely at why discectomy is being done, it becomes clear that fusion is not necessary. The discectomy is performed to relieve the sciatic pain. Discectomy should never be recommended to relieve only low back pain. Therefore, relieving the nerve root irritation by removing the herniated disc fragments should be adequate to alleviate the patient's symptoms.

So why would a fusion be done? Perhaps to prevent potential instability? No studies to date have shown any increase in instability following routine microdiscectomy or limited surgical discectomy. In fact one study that compares the results of the patients undergoing discectomy with and without fusion found the patients who undergo discectomy without fusion fared much better clinically (11). At this time there are no clinical data and certainly no scientific data to suppport the addition of spinal fusion to a routine microdiscectomy or limited surgical discectomy in a patient with a herniated lumbar disc.

REFERENCES

1. Cuckler JM, Bernini PA, Wiesel SW, et al: The use of epidural steroids in the treatment of lumbar radicular pain: A prospective, randomized double blind study. *J Bone Joint Surg* 1985;67A:63–66.
2. Frymoyer JW: Back pain and sciatica. *N Eng J Med* 1988;318:291–300.
3. Haldeman S: Spinal manipulative therapy: A status report. *Clin Orthop* 1983;179:62–70.

4. Kahanovitz N, Viola K, Goldstein T, et al: A multicenter analysis of percutaneous discectomy. *Spine* 1990;15:713–715.
5. Kahanovitz N, Viola K, McCulloch J: Limited surgical discectomy and microdiscectomy: A clinical comparison. *Spine* 1989;14:79–81.
6. McDermott DJ, Agre K, Brim M, et al: Chymodiactin in patients with herniated lumbar disc(s): an open-label, multicenter study. *Spine* 1985;10:242–249.
7. Rosen C, Kahanovitz N, Viola K, et al: A retrospective analysis of the efficacy of epidural steroid injections. *Clin Orthop* 1988;228:270–272.
8. Rutkow IM: Orthopaedic operations in the United States, 1979 through 1983. *J Bone Joint Surg* 1986;68A:716–719.
9. Thomas M, Grant N, Marshall J, et al: Surgical treatment of low backache and sciatica. *Lancet* 1983;2:1437–1439.
10. Weinstein J, Spratt KF, Lehmann T, et al: Lumbar disc herniation: A comparison of the results of chemonucleolysis and open discectomy after ten years. *J Bone Joint Surg* 1986;68A:43–54.
11. White AH, Von Rogou P, Zuckerman J, et al: Lumbar laminectomy for herniated disc: A prospective controlled comparison with internal fixation fusion. *Spine* 1987;12:305–307.
12. Yasuma T, Makino E, Saito S, et al: Histologic development of intervertebral disc herniation. *J Bone Joint Surg* 1986;68A:1066–1072.

8

Spinal Stenosis

Spinal stenosis should be viewed more as a pathologic description than as a distinct pathologic disease entity. In fact spinal stenosis is merely a descriptive term denoting a narrowing or stenosis of the spinal canal. A wide spectrum of anatomic, physiologic, and even genetic abnormalities may result in stenosis of the spinal canal. The most frequent cause of spinal stenosis is the narrowing that often results from long-standing degenerative disease. As the motion segment begins to develop degenerative changes, there are typical anatomic alterations that may ultimately result in spinal canal narrowing. As the aging process causes the collapse and narrowing of the disc space with concomitant facet joint alterations, the neural contents of the spinal canal become victim to encroachment by a variety of anatomic structures.

Anteriorly, the bulging annulus may cause posterior displacement of the dural sac. At the same time a loss in disc height allows for buckling of the ligamentum flavum into the spinal canal both posteriorly and laterally. With more long-standing degenerative change, hypertrophic facet joint spurring, particularly the superior facet, may cause impingement of the exiting nerve root in the lateral recess. Thus with increasing degeneration of the motion segment, there are changes almost circumferentially within the spinal canal that may result in symptomatic spinal stenosis (Fig. 8–1).

Even though degenerative spinal stenosis is by far the most common form of lumbar spinal stenosis, a variety of other spinal abnormalities may result in spinal canal narrowing. Spinal stenosis is a predominant feature of the symptom complex found in a number of the dwarf syndromes. Achondroplasia is probably the best known of these.

In contrast to these more complicated genetic musculoskeletal disorders, isolated spinal canal narrowing due most often to decreased pedicular height may be found in otherwise normal individuals. Fortunately, the incidence of this type of true congenital spinal stenosis is relatively uncommon. Primary or metastatic disease encroaching into the epidural space may result in spinal stenosis. Several metabolic disorders including Paget's disease and acromegaly may result in spinal stenosis. The treatment of patients with these types of stenosis must be determined individually with attention paid to all aspects of the disease process.

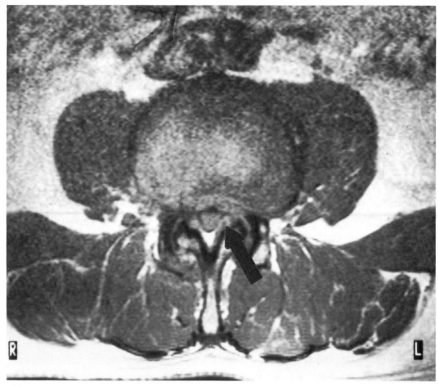

FIG. 8–1. Circumferential degenerative alterations including hypertrophic facet joint changes, buckling of the ligamentum flavum (*arrow*), and disc bulging all contribute to the development of lateral recess and central spinal canal stenosis.

Most patients with degenerative or acquired spinal stenosis become symptomatic in their 60s with the peak presentation early in the eighth decade. However, it is not unusual to find patients with lateral recess stenosis presenting in a transitional age group between ages 50 and 65. Many of the patients with only lateral recess stenosis have not yet developed enough anatomic abnormalities to cause central canal stenosis but have developed enough lateral recess changes secondary to the buckling of the ligamentum flavum and hypertrophic spurring from the superior facets to cause impingement of a single nerve root exiting the lateral recess.

Both lateral recess stenosis and central spinal stenosis are most commonly found at the L4–5 level. Stenosis at the L3–4 level is next most commonly found with L5–S1 usually least involved until marked multilevel involvement occurs. As the interpedicular space continues to widen and the neural contents diminish distally with each exiting nerve root, the L5–S1 space is usually the last of the three distal motion segments to be affected.

The classic history of the patient with spinal stenosis is of ambulatory radicular pain. This type of pain has been called *neural claudication* because of its similarity to vascular claudication. Although radicular pain is the common thread in the history of the patient with spinal stenosis, its anatomic pattern of radiation may be quite variable. Typically the pain may radiate into both lower extremities as would be expected with true sciatic pain. However, it is not unusual for it to be unilateral or radiate only into the buttocks or thigh. The radicular pain may be accompanied by paresthesias or complaints of numbness in the same distribution as the pain. It is also common for the patient to experience a feeling of heaviness in the lower extremities with walking. Although patients with spinal stenosis infrequently have involvement of bladder or bowel function, as with all low back disorders, they should be questioned about the presence of any of these symptoms during the initial interview. Acute urinary or bowel dysfunction should be treated as an emergency as discussed previously.

In contrast to the unilateral radicular pain of a herniated lumbar disc that typically radiates into a predictable dermatomal distribution, the radicular pain pattern in spinal stenosis is much less predictable. However, in patients with only lateral recess stenosis in which a specific root is involved, it is often difficult to distinguish these patients from those with a herniated lumbar disc on the basis of the history alone. What characteristically enables the diagnosis of spinal stenosis is the precipitation of the pain with ambulation and its almost immediate cessation with rest or sitting.

In addition to ambulation, any position that causes extension of the lumbar spine will cause an increase in symptoms. By extending the lumbar spine, the neural elements are further compromised by increased encroachment by the ligamentum flavum, which continues to buckle inward, as well as additional superior facet impingement in the lateral recess. That is why patients have difficulty walking down a hill or flight of stairs. However, with flexion of the spine, the intraspinal dimensions are widened. Activities such as walking up a hill or a flight of stairs are often tolerated well. When questioned about their ability to stand straight, most patients will admit to an increasing propensity to walk in the forward flexed position to avoid pain provoked by standing fully upright. Patients should also be questioned about the speed of onset of symptoms while walking and whether there has been progression of the symptoms over time. With prolonged and severe spinal stenosis the pain may also persist during periods of rest or sitting.

During the physical examination, the physician should first observe the lumbar spine in the standing position. It is most common to find the loss of the normal lumbar lordosis with flattening of the lumbar spine and, frequently, reversal of the lordosis into a mild lumbar kyphosis. The patient should be asked to maximally extend the lumbar spine. This maneuver typically precipitates the radicular pain. The patient should then be asked to forward flex. The pain brought on with extension is usually alleviated immediately with forward flexion.

The vast majority of patients will not exhibit any specific neurologic deficits when examined. The motor and sensory examination is frequently normal in these patients—another distinguishing characteristic from patients with a herniated lumbar disc. It is quite uncommon for these patients to demonstrate any of the positive signs of neural irritability so characteristic of patients with a herniated lumbar disc. The straight leg raising, contralateral straight leg raising, and bowstring tests are almost always negative in patients with spinal stenosis.

The pedal pulses must be present to definitively rule out the possibility of concurrent vascular symptoms. If the pulses in the feet are not palpable, further vascular studies are necessary before arriving at a definitive diagnosis of spinal stenosis.

Patients with spinal stenosis frequently have degenerative disease affecting their peripheral joints. It is important to examine the hips and knees in these patients to avoid misdiagnosing the referred pain of hip or knee arthritis as spinal stenosis.

Plain radiographs will not allow for a definitive diagnosis because of their inability to demonstrate the soft tissue structures. However, the presence of advanced degenerative disease with its associated radiographic findings of disc space narrowing, interlaminar narrowing, and facet hypertrophy suggests the possibility of spinal stenosis (Fig. 8–2). As with a herniated lumbar disc, a definitive diagnosis can be made only with the use of studies illustrating the soft tissue structures, in particular the neural elements.

Because of the more dynamic nature of spinal stenosis, MRI is currently not the diagnostic procedure of choice. Despite its ability to visualize neurologic compression in the sagittal and transverse planes better than CT scanning, at this time MRI still does not provide as much diagnostic information as a myelogram. The use of postmyelography CT is often additionally helpful and should be mandatory in any patient with a complete myelographic block to ensure proper visualization of the intraspinal contents distal to the block. As sophistication and technological advances of MRI continue, it may soon supercede the myelogram as the study of choice in patients with spinal stenosis, but most spinal surgeons at this time prefer the myelogram over MRI in patients with spinal stenosis.

As with any radiographic study, it is imperative that the myelographic abnormalities correlate with the patient's symptoms. Treatment recommendations, particularly those involving surgical intervention, must not be based solely on the radiographic abnormalities. The decision to operate based on the presence of radiographic abnormalities with poor or no clinical correlation will almost certainly result in a large percentage of poor results.

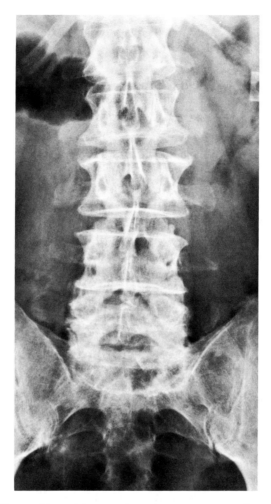

FIG. 8–2. Radiographic evidence of motion segment collapse at the L4–5 level suggests the presence of spinal stenosis. Interlaminar space narrowing, approximation of the spinous processes, and subluxation of the facet joints are radiographic abnormalities typically present in the patient with symptomatic spinal stenosis. However, as with any radiographic abnormality, the radiographic findings must correlate with the patient's symptoms to have clinical relevance.

The treatment of spinal stenosis has received far less attention than that for the patient with a herniated lumbar disc. The causative and precipitating abnormalities are mechanical in nature, and because of the ongoing degenerative process, the space normally afforded the neural contents is no longer present. From a practical standpoint there is virtually no nonsurgical way to restore the space taken away by the degenerative changes. Despite a variety of attempts at active and passive therapeutic modalities, none have been shown to significantly influence the symptoms of spinal stenosis.

The same holds true for medications. Despite a wide array of anti-inflammatory medications, none have been shown to have any long-term effect on improving the symptoms of spinal stenosis. Medications should be viewed as only short-term relief. Avoidance of narcotic medications when possible is wise since most of these patients are elderly and do not tolerate narcotic medications as well as younger individuals. The use of any medication should be dictated by the frequency and intensity of the pain. There is no evidence to suggest that the continuous or prolonged use of any medication will influence the natural history of spinal stenosis. Therefore, it is best to prescribe medication on a PRN basis.

The only nonsurgical method for treating patients with spinal stenosis that has been suggested to alter the long-term course of spinal stenosis is the injection of epidural steroids. Although epidural steroids are widely used to alleviate the radicular pain associated with spinal stenosis, there is a general lack of consensus on its long-term effectiveness. Data suggest that epidural steroid injections may allow short-term relief of symptoms, but there is doubt whether this treatment is any better than placebo treatment on a long-term basis (1,4). Until further clinical data are available, the use of epidural steroids, particularly when used to alter the long-term course of the symptoms, should be done with skepticism despite the fact that their frequent use continues on a widespread basis.

There is little nonsurgical treatment available to the patient with symptomatic spinal stenosis. Surgical intervention is often the only viable treatment modality available to the symptomatic patient. However, patients must be selected carefully. Since there are frequently no abnormal neurologic findings, the decision to operate is often made by the degree of debilitation caused the patient by the pain alone. It is important for the physician to ascertain how much of the patient's normal routine is disrupted by the painful radiculopathy. With no demonstrable neurologic deficits, surgery should be recommended only when the patient is kept from pursuing normal activities because of the spinal stenosis pain.

Preoperative planning is especially important in patients with spinal stenosis. It is critical that only those stenotic levels seen radiographically correlating with the patient's symptoms be operated upon.

Once the exact levels to be decompressed are decided upon, the patient is positioned prone in the knee/chest position to minimize epidural bleeding. The paraspinal muscles are stripped subperiosteally with care being taken not to expose or disrupt the facet joint capsules. Self-retraining retractors allow for the best visualization of the surgical field. All soft tissue is removed from the exposed lamina and ligamentum flavum. The ligamentum flavum is removed with either a scalpel or curette. It is often easiest to enter the spinal canal in the midline near the natural cleft between the right and left ligamentum flavum. In severe spinal stenosis this posterior midline area allows for the safest entrance into the spinal canal.

The remainder of the ligamentum flavum is removed with a Kerrison rongeur and the proximal spinous process removed with a rongeur. At each level, the segmental nerve root should be decompressed adequately on both sides. It is easiest to identify and maintain a normal sense of anatomy by approaching and decompressing each nerve root sequentially. This will allow better visualization of each affected root with less blood loss than doing a multi-level midline decompression and then going back to decompress each nerve root laterally.

It is of the utmost importance that each nerve root be completely freed in the lateral recess. This often requires undercutting of the lateral portion of the ligamentum flavum as well as any osteophytic spurring arising from the superior facet. Visualization and surgical decompression is often easier if performed from the opposite side of the table.

Once the decompression is performed, a final inspection of the nerve roots in the lateral recess is necessary. It is highly unusual to have to perform a facetectomy to adequately decompress a nerve root. Great care is needed to preserve as much facet joint anatomy and, therefore, stability as possible. If an inadvertent total facetectomy is performed, particularly if done so bilaterally, bilateral lateral fusion should be performed to prevent potential instability and iatrogenic spondylolisthesis.

Disc excision is rarely indicated and should only be performed if a true disc herniation is found. The presence of a bulging degenerative disc is not an indication for discectomy and may theoretically allow for potential segmental instability to occur.

Unless the spinal stenosis is caused by a degenerative spondylolisthesis (which will be discussed later), fusion is not necessary. As long as the integrity of the facets are maintained and no sagittal or lateral spondylolisthesis is present, fusion should not be performed.

Drainage of the wound for 24 to 48 hours is necessary to avoid the potential risks of a postoperative epidural hematoma. The patient should be ambulated the evening of surgery or the next day. Postoperatively, the best rehabilitation program is one in which the patients are encouraged to walk as much as possible and gradually return to their normal activities. A steady increase in ambulation will not only increase lower extremity strength but also provide needed aerobic and cardiovascular conditioning so vital for these elderly patients. Once the patients have gone beyond the immediate postoperative period they should be encouraged to increase their activities as tolerated and return to any activity they wish, particularly those they have previously avoided because of the pain.

The best results of spinal stenosis surgery are obtained in patients with symptoms due to central and/or lateral recess stenosis. Good results have ranged from 70 to 85%. Patients with spinal stenosis caused by other etiologies particularly degenerative spondylolisthesis do not fare quite as well postoperatively (2,3). However, in general, most patients do quite well postoperatively with less than 10% of patients having persistent symptoms postoperative and only 5% needing additional surgery at a later date.

REFERENCES

1. Cuckler JM, Bernini PA, Wiesel SW, et al: The use of epidural steroids in the treatment of lumbar radicular pain: a prospective, randomized, double-blind study. *J Bone Joint Surg* 1985;67A:63–66.
2. Hall S, Bartleson JD, Onofrio BM, et al: Lumbar spinal stenosis: Clinical features, diagnostic procedures and results of surgical treatment in 68 patients. *Ann Intern Med* 1985;103:271–275.
3. Nasca RJ: Surgical management of lumbar spinal stenosis. *Spine* 1987;12:809–816.
4. Rosen C, Kahanovitz N, Viola K, et al.: A restrospective analysis of the efficacy of epidural steroids. *Clin Orthop* 1988;228:270–272.

9
Spondylolisthesis

Spondylolisthesis is a term describing a condition in which one vertebra is displaced anteriorly on the vertebra just inferior. Spondylolysis is a condition describing a structural defect of the pars interarticularis. Spondylolisthesis and spondylolysis are present in approximately 7% of the general population. Fortunately, the majority of these patients will never become symptomatic and never require surgical intervention.

The etiology of the spondylolisthesis is best described by the responsible anatomic abnormality. The most common of these are: congenital, isthmic, degenerative, traumatic, and pathologic. The congenital and pathologic types of spondylolisthesis are rare and their diagnosis and treatment will not be discussed here. The most common types of spondylolisthesis are the isthmic and degenerative ones. These two comprise the majority of patients who will present with clinical symptoms caused by a spondylolisthesis.

In younger individuals, isthmic spondylolisthesis is the most common type of spondylolisthesis. For those patients with symptoms, the onset of pain is usually during adolescence or as late as early adulthood. Several types of pars interarticularis abnormalities have been identified that may result in spondylolisthesis. Probably the most common type of isthmic defect is the lytic type in which there is a fibrous defect across the pars (Fig. 9–1). Many of these patients present with an abnormally elongated pars that appears to be more susceptible to fatigue or acute fracture than a more normal-appearing pars. The least common of the isthmic type of spondylosisthesis is one in which an acute fracture of the pars is found.

Despite a vast number of studies attempting to isolate the exact etiology responsible for the pars abnormality, none has been definitively identified in patients with isthmic spondylolisthesis. Although it is unusual to find patients with symptomatic low back pain due to spondylolisthesis prior to adolescence, there are several groups of adolescents and young adults with a higher incidence of this type of pars defect than would normally be expected. The two most recognized groups of high-risk patients are female gymnasts and male football linemen. There is also a higher incidence of spondylolisthesis among family members than would normally be expected as well as in certain Eskimo tribes. Although heredity is a factor in the

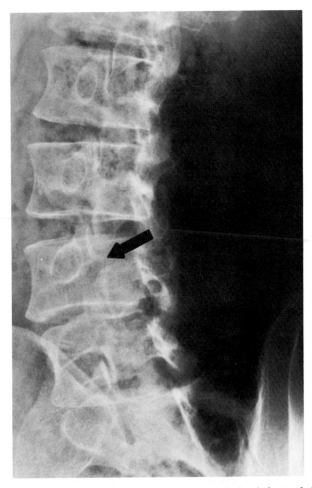

FIG. 9–1. Oblique radiograph revealing a large lytic defect of the L4 pars. Note the disruption of the normal outline of the pars interarticularis (*arrow*).

incidence of lumbar spondylolisthesis, its importance is poorly understood. It is also more common to find an isthmic defect in males than females by an almost 2 to 1 margin. Why these groups tend to have a higher incidence of spondylolisthesis and spondylolysis is not known for sure.

The severity of the slip is best described using a grading system of 0–V. A grade 0 is actually only a spondylolysis but without true listhesis or slippage. Grades I–IV divide the vertebral body into quarters (Fig. 9–2). A 25% or less slip is then referred to as a grade I spondylolisthesis. A slip between 25 and 50% is termed a grade II spondylolisthesis, and so on. A complete slip or spondyloptosis is considered the most severe and referred to as a grade V spondylolisthesis.

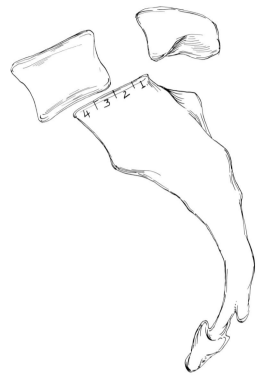

FIG. 9–2. Spondylolisthesis is classified on a grading system denoting progression of the slip from I–IV. Spondyloptosis is described as a complete spondylolisthesis and may be referred to as a Grade V spondylolisthesis.

The vast majority of patients presenting with a spondylolisthesis during childhood and adolescence will never have symptoms of any significance. In fact, one study has found that very few will demonstrate progression of the slip, and even fewer patients will have progression past age 16 (1). Therefore, aggressive surgical treatment in the majority of patients should be avoided as almost all of those with symptomatic spondylolisthesis will improve with time and conservative care.

In those patients who do develop symptoms, the pain is usually not present until the patient reaches his teenage or young adult years. The peak incidence of the onset of pain appears to be at the end of the second decade with a declining incidence thereafter. The pain is most often localized to the lower back. This is particularly true in patients with only a grade I or II slip. Patients with grade III or IV spondylolisthesis may report a higher incidence of radicular pain. It is highly unusual for a patient to present with the acute onset of neurologic loss secondary to a long-standing spondylolisthesis. A thorough search for other intraspinal pathology should be done to insure that no other concomitant abnormality is present.

Patients usually experience an increase in their symptoms with increased activity. Similarly, the low back pain is frequently relieved by rest and restricted activities. As with any low back disorder, patients may experience referred pain in the groin, hips, or thighs, but as always this referred pain pattern must be differentiated from true sciatic pain. Unfortunately, there is often little in the history to distinguish patients with spondylolisthesis from patients with a variety of other etiologic causes of low back pain.

The physical examination often provides information that allows the physician to accurately diagnosis spondylolisthesis. Palpation of the spine may reveal a step-off or defect at the site of the slip. However, patients with very mild spondylolisthesis may not exhibit this physical finding.

The examiner must be careful to realize that the palpable defect is actually present at the level just above the true lytic defect in lytic spondylolisthesis (Fig. 9–3). Thus, in a patient with an L5–S1 spondylolisthesis, because of the lytic defect, the posterior elements of L5 remain posteriorly with the S1 vertebra as the body of L5 slips forward with the more cephalad L4 vertebra. Therefore, the palpable defect in the patient's midline from an L5–S1 spondylolisthesis is actually between the spinous processes of L5 and L4. In contrast, the defect in degenerative spondylolisthesis is palpable at the level of the slip because of the intact pars and only the slippage due to subluxation of the facet joints.

Extremes of forward flexion and/or extension often elicit nonradiating pain at the level of the spondylolisthesis. It is not unusual to have associated hamstring tightness, which further prevents forward flexion. This may also result in posterior thigh pain that should not be confused with true sciatic pain. The exact etiology for the typical hamstring muscle tightness is not understood, although it does not appear to have a neurologic etiology. In severe cases of spondylolisthesis with marked hamstring tightness and secondarily increased lumbar lordosis, significant gait abnormalities may be present due to the shortened stride length as well as the possibility of hip and knee flexion contractures.

Although scoliosis is usually not severe in these patients, there is a higher incidence of idiopathic scoliosis found along with spondylolisthesis than would be expected in the general population. When the scoliosis is detected in an adolescent, treatment should follow the same guidelines for patients with scoliosis in general.

The diagnosis of spondylolisthesis can frequently be suspected by the presence of the above physical findings, but the exact diagnosis must be made radiographically. The spondylolisthesis is best visualized on the standing lateral radiograph. The anteroposterior view may reveal the presence of

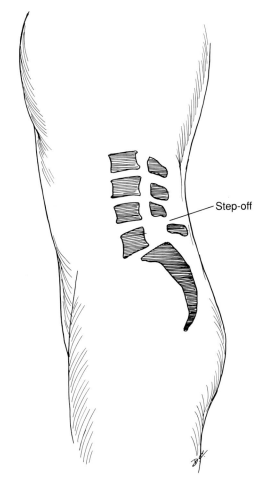

Step-off

FIG. 9–3. The palpable step-off in patients with a lytic spondylolisthesis is actually at the level of the interspace just superior to the actual spondylolytic defect as depicted here in a patient with an L5-S1 spondylolisthesis.

a scoliosis or spina bifida occulta, which are both found more frequently in conjunction with spondylolisthesis than would be expected alone.

The pars abnormalities are best visualized on the oblique radiographs. Infrequently there may be difficulty identifying the pars defect on the oblique radiographs. Oblique tomograms are then often helpful.

It may be impossible to determine whether the patient with the acute onset of pain has suffered a fatigue or even an acute fracture of the pars. In these cases in which the role of acute trauma cannot be determined, bone scintigraphy may be helpful. A normal bone scan is strong evidence that no acute fracture has occurred across the pars and that another source of the acute symptoms should be sought.

The presence of neurologic compression must be identified in patients with sciatic symptoms particularly when surgery has been recommended. Only patients in whom discrete nerve root compression has been demonstrated should undergo surgical decompression. Unfortunately, both MRI and CT scans may be difficult to interpret when attempting to identify nerve root compression at the level of the spondylolisthesis. This is due in large part to the altered anatomy and distortion of the lateral recess on the scans. Too frequently a diagnosis is made of a herniated lumbar disc at the level of a spondylolisthesis when in fact it is only a distortion of the normal disc appearance by the spondylolisthesis.

Myelography is still the procedure of choice in the preoperative evaluation of the patient with spondylolisthesis and sciatic symptoms. Even though an anterior step-off or defect in the anterior column of contrast may be noted, true spinal stenosis or nerve root cutoff must be present to conclusively correlate the sciatic symptoms and the myelographic abnormality. It is extremely rare to find the presence of a herniated disc at the level of the spondylolisthesis. Disc excision at this level should not routinely be performed for fear of inducing additional instability and further progression of the slip.

Most symptomatic patients can be treated successfully without surgical intervention. Patients presenting with their first episode of pain should be treated very much like patients presenting with their first episode of idiopathic low back pain. The initial period of rest should be kept to a minimum prior to slowly returning the patient to normal daily activities. As with idiopathic low back pain, there is little value in the use of any of the passive treatment modalities. Although there have been no definitive studies examining the effects of exercise on the symptoms attributable to a spondylolisthesis, most patients seem to respond well to a reconditioning program, and they improve with time.

The initial treatment should focus on returning the patient to normal activities. The only contraindication to this approach is when the patient is diagnosed as having an acute traumatic fracture of the pars interarticularis. Patients with a traumatic fracture should be treated with immobilization and bracing to maximize the potential for fracture healing. Bracing should be full-time for approximately 12 weeks with a TLSO. It must be remembered that to adequately immobilize the L5-S1 segment, a thigh cuff is needed to gain sufficient distal fixation to control motion at the lumbosacral junction.

Spondylolisthesis due to an acute fracture above L5-S1 may be adequately treated with a standard low-profile thoracolumbosacral orthosis (TLSO). Fabric or elastic corsettes are probably of little value in the treatment of the patient with low back pain secondary to this type of spondylolisthesis. Despite this, many patients obtain a feeling of security with a corsette and claim to feel better with it on.

Patients with long-standing or recurrent low back pain secondary to a spondylolisthesis may not respond as well to a reconditioning program. These more chronic patients may be candidates for bracing or a trial with a body cast. Patients who respond well to the brace or cast and have recurrent symptoms after cessation of the immobilization should be considered good candidates for surgical fusion. Patients who have failed to improve with conservative care, particularly those few patients who have demonstrated progression of their slip, also should be considered for surgical stabilization.

For many years, posterior *in situ* fusion by means of a bilateral-lateral fusion was the universally accepted method of surgical treatment. More recently, a new generation of internal fixation devices for the lumbar spine has now made quite controversial the question of which surgical procedure is appropriate for the patient with spondylolisthesis (3).

It is generally accepted that a grade I spondylolisthesis can be treated quite successfully with an *in situ* bilateral-lateral fusion. Most surgeons agree that a grade II spondylolisthesis can be treated successfully with a bilateral-lateral fusion. However, it is with a grade II and higher spondylolisthesis that the controversy begins.

A variety of internal fixation systems are now available that allow not only rigid internal fixation of the lumbar spine but, in many cases, the ability to reduce the spondylolisthesis. The vast majority of these devices utilize pedicle screw fixation interconnected with either a plate or rod. The most popular of the plate devices are the Steffee and Luque plates. The most widely used rod systems are the Edwards and Cotrel-Dubosset systems. These few are by no means the only systems available and with passing time the inventory of internal fixation devices grows.

Most surgeons agree that the more severe spondylolistheses are better treated with an internal fixation system. Unfortunately, it is not clear whether the increased risk of neurologic compromise in those patients in whom reduction is attempted justifies the use of these devices. The controversy might be easily clarified if there was definitive evidence showing a significantly higher rate of fusion with these devices. Unfortunately, this data is not available at this time. Another perplexing question is, how rigid should the system be to attain the best chance of fusion? There is no clinical evidence at all available to answer this question.

Until more information is available and the long-term results of these internal fixation systems compared to *in situ* fusion are known, the appropriate role of these devices will remain unclear. However, with their ever-increasing popularity, patients with grade III and grade IV as well as some patients with grade II spondylolisthesis are routinely being treated with internal fixation systems (7).

One critical factor must not be overlooked even in the presence of the most rigid of fixation systems: there is no substitute for a meticulous bilateral-lateral fusion. Unless the fusion becomes solid, all internal fixation systems will ultimately fail with time. Therefore, with or without internal fixation, it must always be remembered that success is only measured by the presence of a solid fusion. Without a solid fusion, the chance of success slowly fades.

In general, all patients with internal fixation devices should be rigidly immobilized with a TLSO postoperatively for a minimum of 3–6 months. Patients fused across the lumbosacral junction should have a thigh extension for the first 12 weeks that can then be removed from the TLSO for the remainder of the 6-month period. Patients with an *in situ* fusion should be treated postoperatively the same as patients with internal fixation devices. However, it is not uncommon for patients with a grade I spondylolisthesis to not be rigidly immobilized postoperatively. Unfortunately, there are no data examining the efficacy of postoperative bracing in these patients with respect to increasing the fusion rate. However, the use of bracing in the postoperative period appears to be a small price to pay for a solid fusion after the patient has undergone the inconvenience of surgery.

In contrast to the anatomic abnormality of the pars interarticularis in patients with a lytic spondylolisthesis, there is no such discrete identifiable lesion in degenerative spondylolisthesis. Degenerative spondylolisthesis is a consequence of advanced degenerative changes involving the entire motion segment. As with spinal stenosis, the degenerative changes affect not only the intervertebral disc but subsequently the posterior supporting structures. These anterior and posterior alterations allow for translation of one vertebral body on another with concomitant subluxation of the facet joint (Fig. 9–4). The translation or slip most often occurs in the anterior plain resulting in a spondylolisthesis. However, it is not infrequent to find a retrolisthesis or lateral spondylolisthesis.

The vast majority of the abnormal anatomic changes resulting in a spondylolisthesis are the same as those responsible for spinal stenosis. Therefore, it is not unusual to have a degenerative spondylolisthesis as well as the presence of degenerative spinal stenosis. Patients with degenerative spondylolisthesis are typically in the same or slightly younger age group as those patients with spinal stenosis. It is highly unusual to find a patient with degenerative spondylolisthesis prior to the age of 50. Patients with degenerative spondylolisthesis often present with a significantly higher incidence of neurologic symptoms than patients with lytic spondylolisthesis. This is primarily due to the canal compromising effect of the spondylolisthesis, partic-

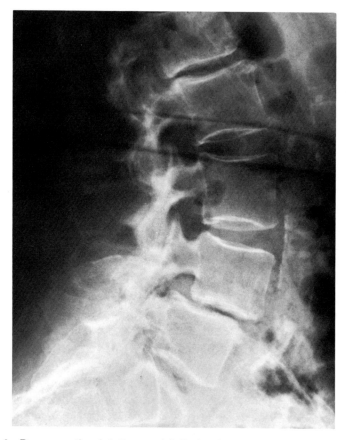

FIG. 9–4. Degenerative L4-5 spondylolisthesis caused by a combination of anterior degenerative disc disease as well as posterior facet joint subluxation. Note the intact pars.

ularly the subluxation of the facet joints resulting in encroachment of the lateral recess. Therefore, it is common for these patients to complain of both significant back and radicular pain characteristic of both spondylolisthesis and spinal stenosis.

As mentioned previously, the step-off is palpable at the level of the spondylolisthesis in contrast to the step-off in lytic spondylolisthesis. Thus, the patient with a degenerative L4–5 spondylolisthesis will have a step-off palpable between the L4 and L5 spinous processes. Otherwise the remainder of the physical examination will be indistinguishable from patients presenting with a lytic spondylolisthesis and/or spinal stenosis depending on the degree of neurologic compression.

The radiographic appearance of degenerative spondylolisthesis is easily distinguished from that of a patient with lytic spondylolisthesis. In the absence of any abnormalities of the pars interarticularis, there is a translation of the vertebra anterior to the vertebra inferiorly. Degenerative spondylolisthesis is most common at the L4–5 level, whereas lytic spondylolisthesis is more common at the L5–S1 level.

Since there is no pars defect that allows elongation of the vertebral ring, it is highly unusual to find a degenerative spondylolisthesis greater than a grade II. Further progression beyond a grade II would require severe degenerative destruction of the facet joint complexes with subsequent severe compromise of the neural canal with significant neurologic involvement. Fortunately this occurs quite infrequently.

In addition to the spondylolisthesis, plain radiographs routinely reveal degenerative changes and subluxation of the facet joints. In patients with sciatic pain with or without neurologic deficit, myelography is the procedure of choice in determining the presence of any lateral recess or central canal stenosis resulting in the pain and symptoms. The presence of true neurologic compression documented on the myelogram is critical prior to recommending surgical decompression. Needless removal of posterior elements may further destabilize an already unstable motion segment. Unfortunately CT scan and MRI should not be relied on solely to recommend neurologic decompression because of the distorted anatomy secondary to the spondylolisthesis.

In contrast to lytic spondylolisthesis, the success of conservative care modalities in the treatment of degenerative spondylolisthesis is rather limited. Passive modalities have no long-term benefit. Exercises have also been of questionable benefit. Anti-inflammatory medications have met with limited success and stronger narcotic medication should not be used on a long-term basis. Rigid bracing may afford temporary relief but most elderly patients tolerate this type of bracing poorly.

Unfortunately, patients with degenerative spondylolisthesis, particularly those with neurologic involvement, may gain relief only with surgical intervention when their symptoms become severe enough. The decision to operate is often quite difficult, particularly in those patients without demonstrable neurological deficits. It is often easier to allow the patient to tell the surgeon when surgery is indicated by his or her inability to perform normal daily activities due to the pain.

In the absence of documented neurologic compression, decompressive laminectomy should not be performed. Only a bilateral-lateral fusion should be performed. Midline posterior fusion should always be avoided particularly in these patients, because of the added risk of developing central canal stenosis at the interspace at the upper limits of the fusion mass. Since the L4–5 level is most often involved in degenerative spondylolisthesis, acceptable results have been obtained with fusion of only the L4–5 level when the L5–S1 segment has been spared significant degenerative changes. This has often been referred to as a "floating fusion."

In those patients without neurologic symptoms, all attempts should be made to definitely ascertain that the back pain is a result of degenerative changes causing the spondylolisthesis. Currently there are no universally accepted diagnostic methods to ascertain this. However, those patients properly selected for spinal fusion must be informed preoperatively that some of their back pain may persist because of the frequency with which other segments of the lumbar spine may be similarly affected by these degenerative changes.

Patients with radicular pain alone but without significant concurrent back pain should undergo appropriate neurologic decompression. It is unclear whether a fusion is necessary as well in these patients. Studies have not conclusively found that patients with degenerative spondylolisthesis and a preponderance of radicular symptoms do any better with only a decompression as they do with a decompression and fusion (2). Unfortunately there are no clear-cut guidelines as to which patients benefit from a concomitant fusion. The need for a fusion should be assessed preoperatively as well as intraoperatively by determining the significance of the decompressive procedure itself with respect to instability. It is probably best to err on the side of fusion when significant doubt arises.

As with other abnormalities in which spinal fusion is indicated, the role of internal fixation, particularly in the reduction of the degenerative spondylolisthesis, is still unclear. With the increasing sophistication of the internal fixation devices, the ability to reduce this type as well as any type of spinal deformity increases. The use of internal fixation to facilitate anatomic reduction must be weighed against its higher morbidity as compared to an *in situ* fusion alone. So far there has been no widely accepted conclusive evidence showing a significantly higher evidence of fusion with internal fixation than without. At this time the decision to use internal fixation devices must be made by the individual surgeon based on his or her surgical skills and perception of the benefits and risks of its use as compared to an *in situ* fusion alone.

An additional type of spondylolisthesis merits consideration. Unfortunately iatrogenic spondylolisthesis occurs with some frequency and is a result of poor surgical planning and a lack of appreciation of the normal vetebral anatomy. Too often a facetectomy is needlessly performed in an attempt to carry out a lateral decompression. As discussed in the section on spinal stenosis, this is rarely necessary.

Postoperatively, the patient may begin experiencing increasing symptoms due to the progressive spondylolisthesis resulting from the previous excessive surgery. It is important for the surgeon to recognize this potential complication and perform a primary fusion before progression of the slip. It is much easier to deal with this potential problem during the inital surgery than to go back and re-operate on an iatrogenic spondylolisthesis in the face of the prior surgical changes.

If untreated primarily and the spondylolisthesis progresses, treatment should be directed at stabilizing and preventing further slip once the diagnosis has been made (6). These patients are probably the best candidates for internal fixation with pedicle screw devices because of the significant loss of stability related to the prior surgery. All efforts should be directed at preventing progression primarily, with reduction a secondary consideration.

For patients with established pseudarthrosis or those at high risk for developing pseudarthrosis, the use of adjunctive electrical stimulation has shown promising results (4,5). Implantation of a direct-current bone growth stimulator has improved the pseudarthrosis and fusion rates in high-risk patients as well as in those patients with established non-union. The use of external electromagnetic pulsing has not gained as wide acceptance and has not had as convincing data presented as to its efficacy compared to the implantable direct-current stimulator.

REFERENCES

1. Frederickson BE, Baker D, McHolick WJ, et al: The natural history of spondylolysis and spondylolisthesis. *J Bone and Joint Surg* 1984;66A:669–707.
2. Herron LD, Trippi AC: L4–5 degenerative spondylolisthesis: The results of treatment by decompressive laminectomy without fusion. *Spine* 1989;14:543–538.
3. Johnson IP, Nasca RJ, Durham WK: Surgical management of isthmic spondylolisthesis. *Spine* 1988;13:93–97.
4. Kahanovitz N, Arnoczky SJ: The use of direct current electrical stimulation to enhance canine spinal fusion. *Clin Orthop* 1990;251:295–299.
5. Kane WJ: Direct current electrical bone growth stimulation for spinal fusion. *Spine* 1988;13:363–365.
6. Sienkiewicz PJ, Flatley TJ: Postoperative spondylolisthesis. *Clin Orthop* 1987;221:172–180.
7. Steffee AD, Sitkowski DJ: Reduction and stabilization of Grade IV spondylolisthesis. *Clin Orthop* 1988;227:82–89.

10

Lumbar Instability

The chapter on lumbar instability could either be the shortest or longest chapter of this book depending on whether it is based on what we truly know about instability or what we think we know. The greatest difficulty in discussing lumbar instability is a complete lack of defining what lumbar instability actually is. This is true not only from a clinical perspective but also from a radiographic perspective as well. Despite a wide array of clinical and theoretical attempts, there has been absolutely no agreement on an objective definition of instability.

The fact that we are unable to agree on a definition of instability makes the measurement or documentation even more difficult and confusing. In the absence of gross or obvious segmental instability, no one has been able to adequately describe a method or a set of variables that accurately establishes lumbar instability. If we accept the fact that there has been no universally accepted definition of instability established nor has there been described a reproducible scientific method of measuring instability, then one can become only further confused over the potential difficulties in trying to treat a patient suspected of having lumbar instability.

Most patients suspected of having lumbar instability present with long-standing symptoms of chronic low back pain. The vast majority of these patients have failed to respond to the conservative care programs that are effective in alleviating pain in most patients. As the patient continues to experience pain, despite attempts by the physician to treat this as best he can, both parties become increasingly frustrated. It is at this point at which all the usual exercise, reconditioning, and other physical therapy treatment fails, that the surgeon begins to tread in very dangerous waters. At the urging of the patient, who is chronically in pain, to do something, no matter what, the physician may begin to consider surgical intervention. After all, he is a spinal surgeon, and, if all else fails, an operation may be able to fix what is broken.

The surgeon now must decide whether to continue with supportive, conservative nonsurgical care or embark on a journey searching for something broken to fix. If he elects the latter path, he has several diagnostic studies from which to choose to validate his claim of lumbar instability.

117

Probably the most widely used radiographic method by which to diagnose lumbar instability is flexion-extension lateral radiographs. These are usually performed with the patient in the standing position. A lateral radiograph is taken of the lumbar spine as the patient actively flexes and extends as far as possible. The amount of translation and angular displacement is measured in an attempt to assess any abnormal motion suggestive or indicative of lumbar instability. Past reports have typically used any angular increase of 10 degrees or more, or translation of 3 mm or more at the L3–4 or L4–5 segments, or 5 mm or more at the L5–S1 level to indicate the presence of lumbar instability. However, more recent studies have shown that abnormal flexion-extension measurements have no statistical correlation with low back pain symptoms (6). In fact, one study examining the interrelationship of observer measurement, quality of the radiograph, and concomitant motion in the planes other than the sagittal has found flexion-extension films highly unreliable in diagnosing instability less than 5 mm (5). Unfortunately, it is the patient with a discrete amount of instability who poses the most difficult diagnostic and therapeutic dilemma. Thus, there is a growing consensus that the long-accepted measurement of instability—flexion-extension radiographs—should no longer be used as the sole basis for surgical intervention because of their high false-positive rate. As more negative reports on the use of standard radiographic studies to diagnose instability appear, it seems more unlikely that these methods will allow reproducible measurements allowing for an accurate diagnosis or definition of instability.

A new radiographic method has been described that has shown some promise. By using dynamic traction and compression, patients with documented instability had a positive correlation with their painful symptoms (1). The same patients undergoing standard flexion-extension radiographs, as expected, did not have the same positive correlation of symptoms and instability. This technique certainly appears more promising than the use of previous standard radiographic studies that in comparison, are relatively useless in detecting clinically relevant instability. However, its use has been limited and further studies and applications are necessary before dynamic flexion-extension radiographs should become widely accepted.

At about the same time that CT discography was becoming more popular, the concept of internal disc disruption also began to be popularized. In fact, the use of CT discography was largely responsible for the concept of internal disc disruption. In theory, internal disruption of the normal concentric disc architecture leads to degenerative changes that manifest themselves clinically as low back pain. A wide variety of grading systems have been proposed to both quantitatively and qualitatively document the extent of the internal disc disruption (3). With the ability to detect even the earliest degenerative changes within the intervertebral disc with MRI, proponents of internal disc disruption can now use this study to support their theory. The noninvasive nature of MRI makes this study an attractive alternative to CT discography with its painful and invasive side effects (4).

The presence of these annular tears and concomitant degenerative changes theoretically causes a degree of segmental instability resulting in long-standing chronic pain unexplained by other standard diagnostic studies. However, opponents of the internal disc disruption theory are quick to point out that the changes seen on both CT discography and MRI are most likely the expected degenerative changes found with the normal aging process. There have been no experimental nor clinical studies that actually demonstrate that this alteration of the normal disc architecture alone is responsible for the painful symptoms. Therefore, it is extremely difficult, from an intuitive viewpoint, to accept this proposed theory of internal disc disruption as the common etiologic factor for patients with chronic low back pain with no other definitive clinical or diagnostic abnormalities.

Thus, it would seem foolish to base a recommendation of surgical fusion to alleviate chronic low back pain on the basis of internal disc disruption diagnosed on either CT discography or MRI. However, because of the chronic nature of the pain, the persistence of the patient insisting that the doctor do something, and the heightening frustration of the surgeon, many of these patients are subjected to surgical intervention for lack of anything else to try. As you might expect, the results are not gratifying. In fact, there are no prospective studies available that document the effectiveness of spinal fusion in alleviating the symptoms due to suspected internal disc disruption. Despite this lack of supportive data, a wide variety of surgical fusion techniques have been proposed to deal with these patients. Anterior interbody fusion, posterior interbody fusion, and posterior bilateral-lateral fusion with and without internal fixation have all been used to treat these patients. The diagnosis of internal disc disruption certainly is one that well describes the presence of degenerative changes within the intervertebral disc. However, until further experimental and clinical data are available, it should never be used alone as evidence to justify lumbar spinal fusion.

Patients with long-standing low back pain who are demonstrated to have significant gross motion on radiographic studies should be treated the same as those patients previously discussed with symptomatic spondylolisthesis. Unfortunately, it is those patients with long-standing low back pain without gross evidence of instability who are so difficult to treat. Fortunately, these patients are in the minority. As discussed above, the diagnosis is often elusive since the identification of true lumbar instability is quite difficult.

Conservative treatment measures should be those of an active nature. Passive modalities alone have no scientific basis in the treatment of these patients with chronic pain and often only serve to reinforce the chronic nature of the patient's pain. Active treatment should be aimed at restoring function, flexibility, and strength. Trunk exercises, aerobic conditioning, and flexibility exercises should all be part of the conditioning program for these patients. Work hardening programs are now gaining widespread popularity. As with back school programs, there is wide variation of programs among the work hardening programs that are becoming popular. This makes assessment of their success quite difficult. However, the early results of a well-supervised overall conditioning program seem to bring new promise to an area that has had little to offer these patients for relief of their chronic pain (2).

As we began this chapter on a note of pessimism, so must we end. Our knowledge of lumbar instability is truly primitive. Until we are able to gain further insight into its true etiology and pathophysiology, we will not be able to fully appreciated its clinical significance. Until we gain this insight, our ability to quantitatively diagnose its presence will also remain primitive. Without this ability to understand the true clinical meaning of lumbar instability and diagnose it accurately, all treatment recommendations, particularly those of an invasive surgical nature, should be approached with the utmost hesitancy.

REFERENCES

1. Friberg O: Lumbar instability: A dynamic approach by traction-compression radiography. *Spine* 1987;12:119–129.
2. Mayer TG, Gatchel RJ, Kishino N, et al: Objective assessment of spine function following industrial injury. *Spine* 1985;10:482–493.
3. Sachs BL, Vanharanta H, Spivey MA, et al: Dallas discogram description: A new classification of CT/discography in low back disorders. *Spine* 1987;12:287–294.
4. Schneiderman G, Flannigan B, Kingston S, et al: Magnetic resonance imaging in the diagnosis of disc degeneration: Correlation with discography. *Spine* 1987;12:276–281.
5. Shaffer WO, Spratt KF, Weinstein JN, et al: The consistency and accuracy of roentgenograms for measuring sagittal translation in the lumbar vertegral motion segment: An experimental model. Presented at the North American Spine Society, Monterey, California, June 10, 1990.
6. Stokes IA, Frymoyer JW: Segmental motion and instability. *Spine* 1987;12:688–691.

11

Postoperative Complications and the Failed Back Syndrome

This chapter is devoted to those patients selected for surgery who have had poor surgical results. The reasons for failure are diverse. However, it must be made clear to all spinal surgeons: "Surgery does not fail, surgeons do!" As we will see in this chapter, the vast majority of surgical failures are due to an error on the part of the surgeon and not the fault of the patient or some unexplained physiologic process.

The most frustrating instance of surgical failure is one in which the preoperative symptoms either did not improve or worsened immediately postoperative. Once again this almost always represents a technical or patient selection error on the part of the surgeon.

By far the most common cause of initial failure is poor patient selection by the surgeon. As enticing as it may seem, surgery is not the cure-all for the large majority of patients with lumbar spine disease. In fact, an acceptable degree of success will be found only when the patient's history and physical findings correlate specifically with the abnormal diagnostic findings. The decision to operate must be based only on these positive and correlative findings. Over the years a variety of grading and rating systems have been devised to quantitate and qualify the patient's chances of surgical success based on the number of positive physical and diagnostic findings. Patients undergoing surgery with weak or no positive physical findings and no confirming diagnostic studies will surely meet with poor results. It can never be overestimated that, no matter how technically skilled the surgeon may be, surgery performed on poorly selected patients will inevitably lead to poor results. That is why the decision to operate must be based solely on the surgeon's objective evaluation of the patient and not on frustration with the inability to cure the patient's symptoms.

After poor patient selection, technical errors account for the second most common cause of initial failure. Surgery performed on the wrong level obviously will result in failure to alleviate the patient's symptoms. It is certainly much easier and less time consuming to obtain an intraoperative radiograph

121

if there is any question over the correct level than having to perform a second operation.

Inadequate decompression is also a common cause of failure, but often much more difficult to prevent than surgery performed at the wrong level. At the time of surgical discectomy, a thorough search should be made for any potentially missed sequestered fragments above or below the level of the disc space as well as laterally through the lateral recess. More commonly encountered than a sequestered disc fragment is the inadequate decompression of lateral recess stenosis. It has been widely recognized that, as patients get older, the possibility of concomitant lateral recess stenosis and a herniated disc increases. Failure to adequately decompress the affected nerve root in the lateral recess will often result in persistent postoperative symptoms. A similar failure to adequately decompress all stenotic neural elements in patients with spinal stenosis, particularly the lateral recess, will also result in a less than optimal resolution of the patient's symptoms. Unfortunately, even with the skill of the most experienced surgeons, there will be cases similar to these that will slip by. The only way to keep their number to a minimum is to consistently insure that each affected nerve root is completely free throughout its course in the spinal canal and lateral recess.

A very small number of patients will sustain acute neurologic trauma at the time of surgery due to a technical mishap. These types of injuries may range from a transient neuropraxia due to excess traction on the retracted nerve root to a complete cauda equina syndrome. The best way to avoid these types of iatrogenic injury is to insure proper surgical exposure with well-controlled hemostasis. Visualization of the affected nerve root is critical during the surgical procedure in order to avoid these catastrophic injuries. Careful retraction and visualization of the nerve root should virtually eliminate the possibility of nerve root avulsion or dural laceration.

Repair of all dural tears primarily will avoid the possibility of postoperative infection and spinal fluid fistula formation. Careful hemostasis and appropriate postoperative drainage should be used to avoid the possibility of a postoperative hematoma and subsequent cauda equina syndrome. Progressive postoperative neurologic deficit warrants immediate diagnostic myelography and/or MRI with appropriate timely treatment to avoid permanent neurologic loss. The vast majority of these technical complications resulting in the more common postoperative and operative complications are easily avoided if strict adherence to proper surgical technique is maintained. Unfortunately, this is not always the case.

A second group of patients with the failed back syndrome do quite well immediately postoperative. These patients have complete or satisfactory relief of their symptoms lasting weeks to months before their previous symptoms recur or new ones present. Patients presenting with increasing low back pain ranging from 10 days to several weeks postoperative should be suspected of having a disc space infection or discitis. Patients often complain of progressive nonradiating pain that is not relieved completely by rest. Most often there is no true sciatic pain initially. Percussion of the spine typically elicits exquisite tenderness. The patient may or may not have systemic symptoms such as fever or chills. Although the laboratory studies may be normal early on, the erythrocyte sedimentation rate (ESR) is almost always elevated, even in the earliest stages of discitis. Radiographically, the affected disc space is narrowed. However, at the onset of symptoms, no radiographic changes may be present. The most sensitive study to detect the presence of infection is bone scintigraphy (Fig. 11–1). A positive bone or a gallium scan is strong evidence of the presence of a disc space infection. Unfortunately, there is no definitive evidence that intraoperative and immediate postoperative antibiotics are useful. In fact, patients with diagnosed discitis often do as well with antibiotic treatment as without, although antibiotic treatment should be instituted once a definitive organism has been obtained. This often requires needle biopsy of the disc space to obtain a specimen for diagnosis. Unfortunately, despite repeated attempts, an organism is often never found. It is specifically these patients for whom antibiotic treatment is of questionable value.

Patients who have had relief of their symptoms and present with similar radicular symptoms months to years postoperative should be suspected of

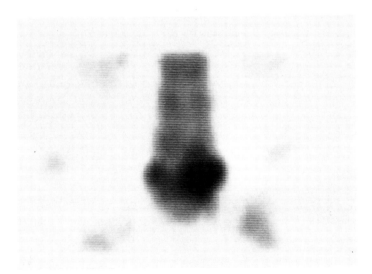

FIG. 11–1. Bone scan illustrating markedly increased uptake 6 weeks following surgical discectomy. Needle biopsy revealed staphyloccus aureus as the source of infection.

having a recurrent disc herniation. Despite the skill or expertise of the surgeon, there will always be at least 3–5% of these patients who will experience a recurrence of their herniation. The recurrence typically occurs at the same level and side as before. Occasionally these patients may have a disc herniation at another level. This should probably be considered a new clinical problem and not a recurrence.

These patients present with the characteristic history and physical findings similar to those patients who are experiencing a disc herniation for the first time. Some patients may appear either more accepting or more anxious and frightened when presenting with recurrent symptoms than they did at their first episode. Often the anxiety and fear may cause exaggeration of the symptoms out of proportion to what one would expect. As always, correlation of the history and physical findings with the abnormal diagnostic studies is of the utmost importance prior to recommending definitive treatment, particularly surgical intervention.

Until recently the most widely used diagnostic study in patients with previous surgery was the water soluble myelogram followed by a contrast-enhanced CT scan. This provided the best possibility of differentiating post-operative epidural scarring from an actual recurrent disc herniation. With the advent of the gadolinium-enhanced MRI, this study appears to be becoming the study of choice in the diagnosis of recurrent disc herniation (Fig. 11–2).

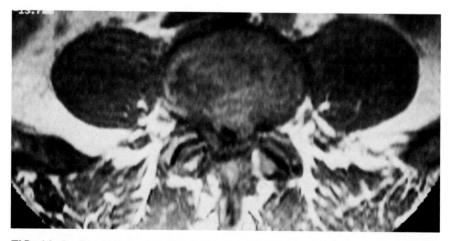

FIG. 11–2. Discrete areas of localized epidural scarring are seen with gadolinium enhancement, but the large avascular recurrent disc herniation was responsible for this patient's recurrent radicular pain and not the epidural scarring.

It is quite common for patients to be told that their pain is due to post-operative scarring. It is virtually impossible for postoperative scarring to be the true cause of sciatic pain in the immediate postoperative period since there has been no time for significant scarring to form. It must be remembered that all patients undergoing back surgery will have some degree of postoperative epidural scarring. Rarely is the epidural scar the actual cause of the pain.

Patients diagnosed with a recurrent disc herniation should be treated as if this were their first episode. Appropriate conservative care as discussed previously should be recommended for a minimum of 4–6 weeks in the absence of significant or progressive neurologic involvement. Only after the patient has failed to improve within this period of time should surgical discectomy be considered and only after the diagnostic studies have definitively confirmed the clinical findings.

Surgery should address the abnormal findings delineated on the myelogram, CT scan, or MRI. Of primary importance is the alleviation of any recurrent disc herniation and degenerative or lateral recess stenosis. In the majority of patients with a preponderance of sciatic pain rather than back pain, adequate nerve root decompression will most often give satisfying relief of symptoms. However, in those patients with a significant component of back pain as well as sciatic symptoms, the role of fusion remains controversial. Although lumbar fusion is frequently performed at the time of decompression for a recurrent disc herniation, there are no studies that have found that patients with fusion do any better than patients without. In view of the lack of definitive evidence that fusion improves the clinical success of patients undergoing surgery for recurrent disc herniation, it should not be routinely performed at the time of recurrent disc excision. Its use should be reserved for those patients in whom gross iatrogenic or degenerative instability is present.

Patients with recurrent symptoms, despite the severity, should never be considered surgical candidates unless there is an identifiable anatomic lesion responsible for their symptoms. Regardless of the significance of the pain or the frustration of the patient and surgeon, without an identifiable lesion, exploratory surgery is never, ever indicated. Re-operation in an area of epidural scarring and possible arachnoiditis may initially result in temporary relief. However, with great predictability, these patients will soon experience a recurrence of pain that often becomes worse than it had been preoperatively. Therefore, it cannot be overemphasized that surgery must be reserved only for those patients with documented pathology correlating to their symptoms. Less stringent selection criteria will end in very poor results and very unhappy patients.

For those patients found not to be candidates for surgery, alternative non-

surgical care may be difficult to formulate, with less than satisfactory results. Initially patients with non-operative failed back syndrome should be
treated much the same as other patients with the acute onset of pain. Many
of these patients will respond as expected. However, there will remain a few
patients with persistent pain who become frustrating therapeutic dilemmas.
This is particularly true for those patients with sciatic pain that appears to be
due to excessive epidural scarring or arachnoiditis. Patients not responding
to the usual type of initial conditioning and treatment may then require more
intensive multidisciplinary treatment. Psychological testing, vocational rehabilitation, pain management as well as traditional physical therapy may be
needed to address the complex nature of these patients' pain and symptoms.

This type of approach is best performed with a multidisciplinary team of
health care professionals specializing in the care of patients with chronic
nonsurgical pain. A wide variety of pain programs are now available to deal
with this type of patient. It is extremely important when choosing a program
of this type that only those programs that include active (as opposed to
passive) treatment be used. As with all types of back pain, passive modalities such as massage, ultrasound, trigger point injections, and the like have
no therapeutic role for these patients. Use of these passive modalities often
serves only to reinforce the chronic pain syndrome manifested by these patients. It is imperative that these patients be made to take control of their
lives and become as active in their treatment programs as possible. Unfortunately, because of the diverse nature of these pain programs, there are no
clear-cut data available to universally support their long-term effectiveness.
However, for lack of a better alternative, their selected use for the proper
patient seems to be the best alternative for functional recovery.

For those patients previously not considered to be surgical candidates,
recent improvements in surgically implanted epidural electrical stimulators
have shown early clinical success. Even though their early success needs to
meet the test of time, as with any surgical procedure, patient selection appears critical. These epidural implants should be used only for patients with
sciatic pain and not for patients with primarily low back pain. All use of
narcotic medication should be stopped prior to consideration for surgical
implantation. Although their recent technologic advance appears to make
this a relatively safe surgical procedure, its long-term effectiveness needs to
be established before widespread use can be recommended.

12

Other Causes of Low Back Pain

There is a common misconception among patients that back pain may be caused by osteoporosis. Postmenopausal females frequently visit a doctor for idiopathic low back pain and the first question asked is "How much osteoporosis do I have?" This concept of pain caused by the osteoporosis is probably the result of the aggressive advertising of the calcium supplement manufacturers. It is important for patients to understand that it is not the osteoporosis that is primarily responsible for their pain. In fact it is secondary to the structural changes caused by the progressive osteoporosis on the normal alignment of the spine that result in the painful alteration of the normal motion segment mechanics.

In postmenopausal and elderly patients, minor trauma or loading of the spine may exceed the fracture threshold of the osteoporotic vertebrae resulting in a vertebral microfracture. These microfractures may be acutely painful but may fail to show any radiographic deformity on plain radiographs. Bone scintigraphy may be more successful at detecting these small fractures.

Increased spinal loading in combination with more advanced osteoporosis in the face of a lowered fracture threshold will then lead to a radiographically apparent compression fracture (Fig 12–1). These may be found singly or at several levels depending on the degree of the osteoporosis and the significance of the applied load. It is not uncommon to have acute fractures adjacent to older healing compression fractures in severely osteoporotic individuals. Unfortunately, once the osteoporosis has advanced to this stage, it is difficult and sometimes virtually impossible to reverse the osteoporosis to the point at which the fracture threshold is improved. The use of calcium supplements, vitamin D, fluoride, hormonal therapy, and exercise have all been shown to play a role in preventing the progression of osteoporosis, but significant reversal of severe osteoporosis is not yet readily attainable.

The treatment of a symptomatic compression fracture is one of reassurance and emotional support. Attempts at bracing are usually unsuccessful because of the elderly patient's intolerance of rigid bracing with a TLSO. Less rigid bracing may afford some symptomatic relief but offers relatively

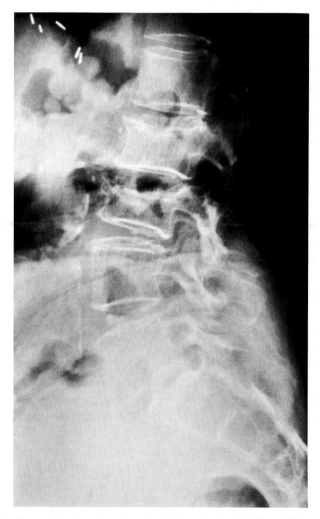

FIG. 12–1. Once the fracture threshold has been lowered by progressive osteoporosis, minor trauma may often result in the characteristic compression fracture seen acutely at L3 as well as the healed fracture at L2.

little rigid immobilization. Patients should understand that, as with fractures of any bone, their compression fractures will need time to heal. Most routine osteoporotic compression fractures heal within 2–3 months with gradual diminution of pain.

Late kyphotic deformity may occur following a significant solitary compression fracture. However, more common than developing a kyphotic deformity is the reversal of the normal lumbar lordosis with multiple smaller compression fractures. The pain is due in large part to subluxation and alteration of the normal facet joint articulations as well as alteration of the entire motion segment alignment. Unfortunately, there is little definitive treatment for the patient with this type of mechanical pain due to multiple osteoporotic compression fractures. As stated above, these patients tend to tolerate rigid bracing poorly and less than rigid immobilization offers little symptomatic relief. Advising the patients to remain active, to exercise daily, and to control the pain with nonsteroidal, non-narcotic pain medication is all that is frequently available for these patients.

Surgery is rarely indicated unless there has been neurologic compression secondary to the collapse and deformity. Attempts at correcting the kyphosis in a neurologically normal patient have not met with great success. The osteoporosis and the age of these patients is often not compatible with performing major reconstructive spinal surgery.

When diagnosing and treating an elderly patient with what is suspected of being an osteoporotic compression fracture, it is always important to keep in mind the possibility of a primary or metastatic tumor causing the fracture. It is often difficult to differentiate early tumorous involvement of a vertebral body from an osteoporotic compression fracture. Occasionally the cortical margins of the vertebral body are lost and a pedicle may be eroded in a patient with a vertebral tumor. These changes are not present with an osteoporotic compression fracture. Unfortunately, bone scintigraphy is usually positive in both instances and is not helpful in differentiating the two. CT scanning and MRI are probably the best studies by which to identify an invasive lesion, particularly if there is soft tissue extension of the tumor (Fig. 12–2). Evidence of bony erosion and soft tissue invasion is strong evidence of a vertebral tumor.

The most common primary malignant tumor to affect the lumbar spine is the solitary plasmacytoma (3). Chordoma is also found in the lumbar spine but with much less frequency. A variety of other primary malignant bone tumors have been reported to affect the lumbar spine but with significantly much less frequency than plasmacytoma or chordoma. The most common benign bone tumors affecting this region of the spine are the benign giant cell tumor, osteoid osteoma, osteoblastoma, osteochondroma, and eosinophilic granuloma. Most malignant tumors are found anteriorly in the vertebral body while benign tumors have a proclivity for the posterior elements. Primary intradural and rarely metastatic intradural tumors may present the same symptoms as those benign and malignant tumors principally affecting the vertebra.

With advancing age, metastatic tumors far outnumber the cases of primary bone tumors affecting the spine. Virtually any malignant tumor can metastasize to the lumbar spine but multiple myeloma, renal, prostrate, breast, and lung are some of the more common primary tumors. Most pa-

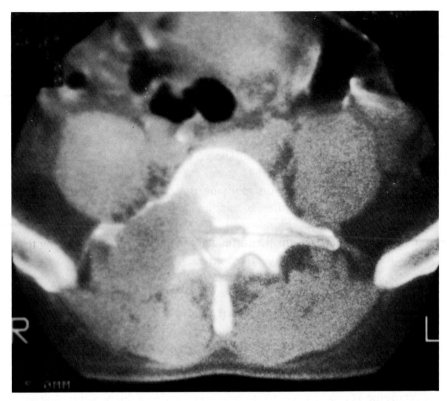

FIG. 12–2. CT scan of a patient presenting only with low back pain. Plain radiographs were normal except for the absence of the pedicular cortex on the AP radiographs. Metastatic carcinoma was diagnosed at open biopsy.

tients present with complaints of localized back pain that is constant and unremitting. Only one quarter of patients will present with sciatic pain; a significantly higher percentage of patients with malignant tumors will have neurologic symptoms than will those patients with benign tumors. Definitive diagnosis is made by histologic identification of the tumor by either closed or open biopsy. Treatment should take into account the sensitivity of the tumor to available chemotherapy and radiation therapy, the presence of any mechanical instability, neurologic deficits, and the long-term prognosis of the patient.

During pregnancy, a great number of women experience low back pain. This is particularly common during the last 4 months of pregnancy. Although many of these women also complain of sciatic pain during pregnancy, it is rare for patients to develop a true lumbar disc herniation (2). The exact etiology for the low back pain is not clear. There is no evidence that the mother's weight gain, baby's weight, or prior pregnancy has any affect on the incidence of low back pain in pregnant women. Treatment should consist of the routine exercise program usually prescribed for patients with idiopathic low back pain. Surgery should never be contemplated unless there are severe or progressive neurologic deficits.

Probably the only thing more difficult than spelling coccygodynia is treating it. Outside of the rare case of pain caused by tumor or infection involving the coccyx, the true etiology of the pain is unknown. Plain radiographs and bone scintigraphy are usually adequate to rule out the possibility of acute fracture, tumor, or infection. The vast majority of patients will have no distinctive radiographic findings.

Treatment is best focused on relieving direct pressure over the coccyx during sitting. This is most often accomplished by having the patient sit on a foam doughnut-shaped cushion. Local steroid injections are frequently performed in the area of the pain. Unfortunately, there are no data showing that this type of treatment has any effect on the long-term outcome. Surgical excision as a last-ditch effort to relieve the pain has met with very mixed results. At this time it is difficult to recommend surgical excision when the surgeon is not sure why or what he is excising.

The most recently described abnormality to affect the lumbar spine has been called lumbar spine osteolysis (1). Patients typically present with increasing motion segment instability while radiographically demonstrating increasing osteolysis of the affected vertebrae. Its etiology is not known but this syndrome is found most commonly after wide decompressive surgery. Biopsy specimens are normal as are bacteriological cultures and the ESR. The treatment should be directed at preventing further instability and collapse, as well as decompressing any neurologic compression. Until new information as to the exact etiology of lumbar spine oesteolysis is available, prevention of this disorder is unlikely.

REFERENCES

1. Bradford DS, Gotfried Y: Lumbar spine osteolysis: An entity caused by spinal instability. *Spine* 1986;11:1013–1019.
2. Fast A, Shapiro D, Ducommun EJ, et al: Low back pain in pregnancy. *Spine* 1987;12:368–371.
3. Weinstein J, Mclain RF: Primary tumors of the spine. *Spine* 1987;12:843–851.

13
Risk Factors

Throughout this book we have repeatedly voiced frustration over the inability to determine the exact etiologic cause for the symptoms in the majority of patients with low back pain. This obviously makes the exact diagnosis and treatment of many of these patients difficult. Despite this persistent obstacle, we are achieving much greater success in predicting which patients are at greater risk among the general population for developing low back pain and for those patients experiencing symptoms who will likely not improve.

Certainly the most widely recognized risk factor for delayed recovery is whether the patient was injured at work (2). (Table 13–1) However, the presence of a Worker's Compensation claim does not necessarily predict disaster. Worker's Compensation patients with sedentary jobs tend to recover more quickly and with less long-term disability than patients with more strenuous jobs. In fact there is a direct relationship between the risk of prolonged back pain and the more physically demanding the job. Patients involved in repetitive bending and lifting, particularly involving heavy objects, do more poorly over the long term. The addition of chronic vibration as may be found in driving a truck also predisposes the patient to a less favorable outcome. In addition, any job that requires a significant amount of repetitive carrying, pushing, and pulling carries an increased risk of the worker's developing and continuing with low back pain once it begins.

In general, patients with Worker's Compensation (and in particular blue-collar workers) fare more poorly when treated for low back pain than other patients. This is even more true with patients undergoing surgery (3). Blue-collar Worker's Compensation patients take longer to return to work following disc surgery, are out of work longer preoperatively, have more significant postoperative signs and symptoms, return less frequently to the same job, and, overall, return to work less than a comparable group of sedentary Worker's Compensation patients. Even though the sedentary patients had better postoperative results than the blue-collar Worker's Compensation patients neither group did nearly as well postoperatively as a comparable group of blue-collar and sedentary private insurance patients not injured on the job. Therefore, it is of the utmost importance that very selective diagnostic criteria be met prior to performing surgery on a blue-collar Worker's Com-

TABLE 13-1. Job-related risk factors

Blue Collar
    Repetitive bending, lifting, pushing, pulling
    Vibration
    Heavy lifting
Job dissatisfaction
Poor work history
Litigation—attorney
Prior disability
Receiving disability payments
Nearing retirement age
Acute injury

pensation patient. It is also wise to inform the patient, as well as the insurance carrier, preoperatively that even with optimal results there is a very significant chance that this patient will not be able to return to blue-collar labor postoperatively. In this way preoperative vocational counseling can be begun to avoid unnecessary and often frustrating postoperative delay in returning the patient to a productive lifestyle.

There are other factors that additionally contribute to an increased incidence of disability (Table 13–1). Patients not satisfied with their occupation will return to work less frequently than those patients who enjoy their occupation. Patients who view their occupation as the cause of their low back pain will also return to work less frequently. Any patient with a Worker's Compensation claim who also has an attorney pursuing an active claim will not do as well while the attorney is still litigating the case as when the case has been settled (5).

Obviously patients receiving disability payments, as well as patients who have been disabled in the past, will do more poorly than self-employed patients receiving no disability payments. The same increased probability of disability holds true for patients experiencing symptoms as the time for their retirement nears. The same is true for patients with multiple episodes of previous low back pain severe enough for hospitalization and patients with a generally poor work history or frequent job changes with time lost from work.

Patients injured acutely tend to have a higher risk for disability than those patients injured insidiously over a longer period of time. Even though the incidence of low back pain in the general population decreases into the fifth and sixth decades, there is an increased risk of disability in older patients injured at work than in younger patients. This may be due, in part, to a combination of job boredom and dissatisfaction as well as a desire for early retirement.

A variety of risk factors independent of insurance or Worker's Compensation status may also predict a poor clinical outcome and are often associated with prolonged disability and chronic pain (Table 13–2). These risk factors, if present in conjunction with the above job-related risk factors, are predictive of a very poor prognosis.

A large variety of psychological studies have been used to document any number of psychological disturbances predictive of prolonged disability and chronicity. Probably the best known of these are the hypochondriasis and hysteria scales on the Minnesota Multiphasic Personality Inventory (MMPI). Depression and somatization of symptoms documented on any number of psychological tests likewise are predictive of an increased risk of disability. Similar defects in the normal coping mechanisms are also a poor prognostic sign. Patients with any previous chronic pain behavior such as recurrent headaches or neck pain are at high risk of developing chronic low back pain. Overall, patients who are emotionally and mentally healthy have a much lower likelihood of developing chronic and disabling low back pain than those patients with any psychological disturbances.

A variety of studies have attempted to correlate body habitus, particularly obesity, with the incidence and severity of low back pain. Unfortunately, the results of these studies are not conclusive in identifying any body habitus characteristic of an increased incidence of back pain. In contrast, there is a very positive correlation with a decreased incidence of disability and recurrence in patients who are physically fit. In fact there is preliminary evidence that pre-employment strength testing may allow for screening of prospective blue-collar workers with a higher-than-expected likelihood of experiencing disabling low back pain (1). Although these reports are promising, long-term and more extensive data are needed before pre-employment strength testing should be widely accepted.

Increased use of alcohol tends to have an overall risk of disability that may not be specific to low-back-related disorders. Smoking, however, seems to specifically increase the risk of low back pain and disc disease (4).

TABLE 13-2. General risk factors

Psychological impairment
    Minnesota Multiphasic Personality Inventory (MMPI)—hypochondriasis, hysteria, depression
    Altered coping mechanisms
    Somatization
Previous psychosomatic illness
Poor physical fitness
Alcoholism
Smoking
Prior hospitalizations for back pain

Physiologic studies have shown that smoking impairs the blood supply to the vertebral endplate and thereby decreases the nutrition of the intervertebral disc. Further clinical and experimental studies are needed for additional clarification, but there appears to be a decisive correlation between smoking and an increased risk of developing low back pain.

It should be obvious in this rather lengthy and ever-growing list of low back pain risk factors that there is more than meets the eye when interviewing and examining a patient with low back pain. These risk factors should be kept in perspective and used appropriately. First and foremost in arriving at a diagnosis and formulating a treatment plan is to base your conclusions on the clinical impressions derived from the history, physical examination, and diagnostic studies. It is then appropriate to temper any unrealistic outcome or treatment predictions by the identifiable risk factors. Any inappropriate prejudice toward the patient by considering these risk factors primarily may eventually and tragically result in the misdiagnosis and inappropriate treatment of many curable low back disorders.

REFERENCES

1. Bierring-Sorenson F: Physical measurements as risk indicator for low back trouble over a one-year period. *Spine* 1984;9:106.
2. Frymoyer JW, Cats-Baril W: Predictors of low back pain disability. *Clin Orthop* 1987;221:89–97.
3. Kahanovitz N, Viola K, et al.: A multicenter comparative analysis of workmen's compensation and private patients undergoing surgical discectomy. Presented at the International Society for the Study of the Lumbar Spine April 14, 1988, Miami, Fla.
4. Kelsey JL, Githens PB, O'Connor T, et al.: Acute prolapsed intervertebral disc: an epidemiologic study with special reference to driving automobiles and cigarette smoking. *Spine* 1984;9:908–913.
5. Trief P, Stein N: Pending litigation and rehabilitation outcome of chronic back pain. *Arch Phys Med Rehabil* 1985;66:95.

Subject Index